PRAISE FOR TEN PATHWAYS

This heartfelt, smart, and practical book will help you feel better from the very first page. Fleur Chambers has a remarkable gift for offering super-effective ideas and tools in a warm, down-to-earth, and encouraging voice. Plus it's just beautiful. This is a gem.

Rick Hanson PhD, author of *Buddha's Brain: The Practical Neuroscience of Happiness, Love, and Wisdom*

Your go-to guide for good days, bad days and everything in between. Fleur has an amazing ability to reframe what it means to be happy and drop her readers into gratitude. Whether you've experienced chronic pain or not, the ten pathways aren't a quick fix, but a total mindset reset. Every page delivers a big dose of healing! This book is a gift!

Amy Molloy, author of *Wife Interrupted*

Life can be painful and messy. But — according to Fleur Chambers — joy and vitality can be found in the midst of the mess. In this beautifully designed book, written with humour and wisdom, Fleur shows us how. Equal parts whimsical and sensible, reassuring and wise, it will make you feel better even if it just sits on your bedside table!

Matthew Young, director, Melbourne Meditation Centre

Fleur's book is a wonderful resource for anyone who is curious about how mindfulness can help with any kind of pain. Full of practical, thoughtful ideas, as well as Fleur's personal journey, this engaging and beautiful book will make you feel that you're sitting in the room with a kind and supportive friend.

Kate James, author of *Change Your Thinking to Change Your Life*

Ten Pathways by Fleur Chambers is a sanctuary for your soul. Fleur has delivered a place for us to retreat into when we need support on our journey. I am in love with this book and am honoured to publish it. *Ten Pathways* is Fleur's gift to humanity, it makes the world a better place.

Karen Mc Dermott, publisher, author, TEDx speaker

FOR MORE PRAISE, PLEASE VISIT
THE HAPPY HABIT WEBSITE.

(www.thehappyhabit.com.au)

Ten Pathways

We are taught to avoid pain — physical, emotional, psychological, or mental. There's an expectation that we will push it aside or squash it down so we can continue to strive towards the 'good life' — an imaginary place free of disappointment, regret, insecurity, or any other uncomfortable emotion.

Imagine if you woke up tomorrow, your whole body screaming in pain, and according to all the experts, there was no solution ... except to find acceptance. This is what happened to Fleur Chambers, who faced a diagnosis with no cure and a crossroads moment: she could either see herself as a victim or lean into the deeper lessons her pain was teaching her — and use these hard-won insights to help people around the world.

Fleur Chambers is a multi-award-winning, internationally recognised meditation teacher and creator of *The Happy Habit* app. Her offerings have been downloaded two million times in forty different countries.

In this uplifting and life-changing guide, Fleur reveals her ten pathway framework for redefining happiness in a way which will allow you to safely meet your challenges, access their wisdom, and embrace all of life — including the parts which caught you by surprise!

Fleur's gentle style combined with her ability to laugh at herself has encouraged people across the globe to befriend themselves and their lives. Come take a walk to a new version of happiness.

Ten Pathways

A FRAMEWORK FOR REDEFINING HAPPINESS

FLEUR CHAMBERS

www.thehappyhabit.com.au

Copyright © Fleur Chambers
First published in Australia in 2022
by KMD Books
Waikiki, WA 6169

All rights reserved. No part of this book may be used or reproduced by any means, graphic, electronic, or mechanical, including photocopying, recording, taping or by any information storage retrieval system without the written permission of the copyright owner except in the case of brief quotations embodied in critical articles and reviews.

Because of the dynamic nature of the Internet, any web addresses or links contained in this book may have changed since publication and may no longer be vaild. The views expressed in this work are solely those of the author and do not necessarily reflect the views of the publisher and the publisher hereby disclaims any responsibility for them.

This book is not intended as a substitute for the medical advice of physicians. The reader should regularly consult a physician in matters relating to their health and particularly with respect to any symptoms that may require diagnosis or medical attention.

Illustration and cover design by Sarah Hankinson
Book design by Bree Hankinson
Editing by Amy Molloy

 A catalogue record for this work is available from the National Library of Australia

National Library of Australia Catalogue-in-Publication data:
Ten Pathways/Fleur Chambers

ISBN: 978-0-6454374-5-4 (Hardback)
ISBN: 978-0-6454374-6-1 (Paperback)
ISBN: 978-0-6454374-7-8 (Ebook)

To Tom, Gabe, and Dash,
my most compelling reasons to linger in the present.

CONTENTS

Introduction	....	1
Awareness	....	13
Compassion	....	33
Perspective	....	61
Gratitude	....	89
Calm	....	115
Connection	....	137
Purpose	....	161
Vitality	....	183
Confidence	....	205
Acceptance	....	223
Epilogue	....	251
References	....	261
Acknowledgements	....	266

INTRODUCTION

Life beyond the resistance

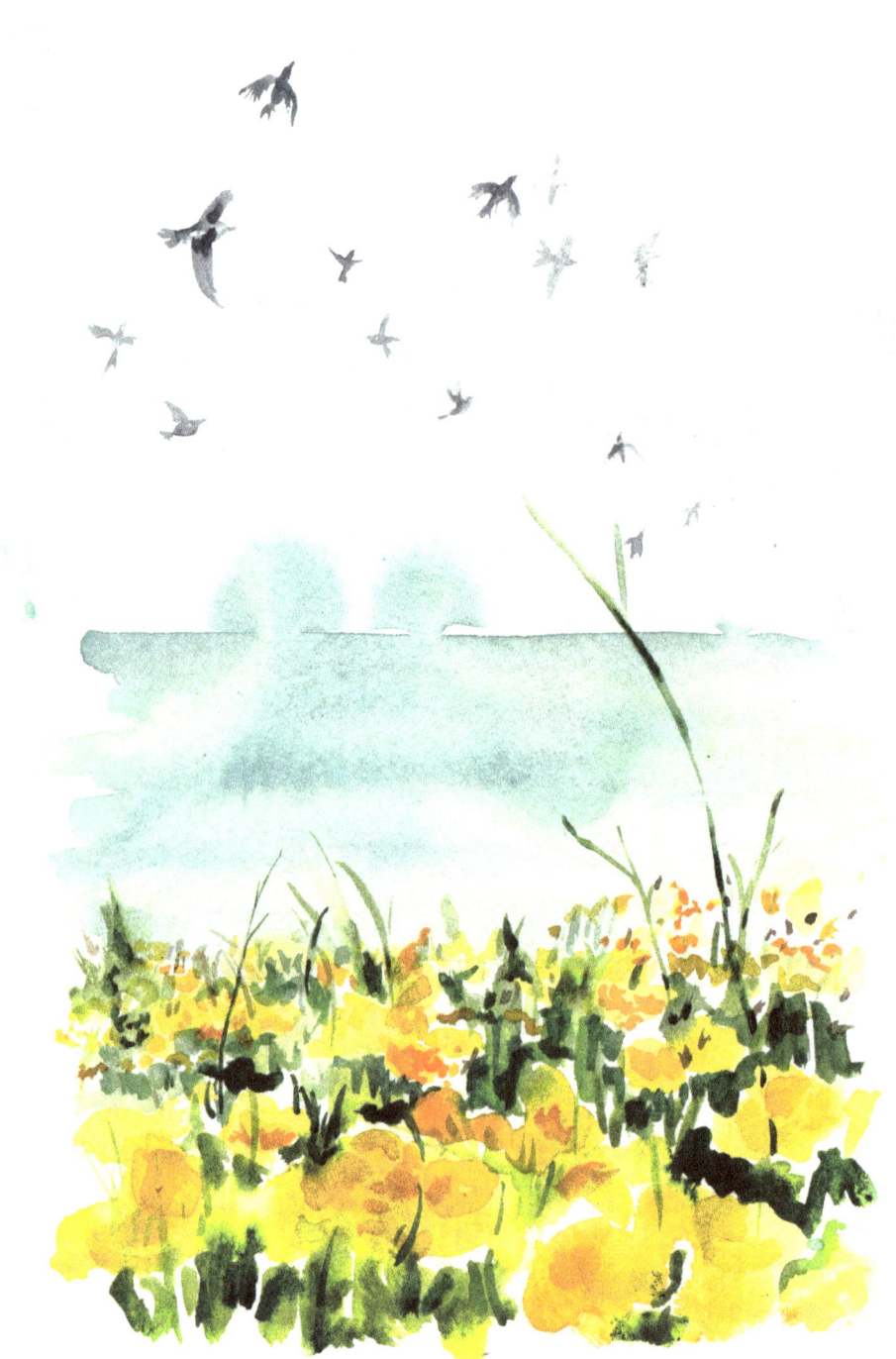

INTRODUCTION

I don't want to get to the end of my days and realise I've hurried through huge parts of my life, thinking that only the good times matter. Do you?

I'm a mother, wife, daughter, sister, and friend. I'm a meditation teacher, app creator, philanthropist, and student of life. I enjoy the ocean, but I'm scared to go too deep. Birds bring me joy, but not up too close. I love, and I worry. I'm both brave and a little afraid. I guess I'm full of contradictions. Aren't we all?

I believe happiness is possible, even amidst the setbacks, regrets, and disappointments of adult life. I trust that our challenges offer gifts in the form of greater resilience, purpose, and insight.

This is me: a happy person who also accepts that life doesn't have to look perfect. An optimist. A glass-half-full type of woman. Or it *was* me, until the pain began — a chronic cycle of physical pain, which would span a seven-year period of my life, plunging me into moments of darkness.

This darkness would also give me many gifts, some of them totally unexpected, and eventually help me to discover what real happiness feels like. A happiness you can find, not in the absence of challenges, but in living wholeheartedly alongside them.

I spent much of my late thirties and early forties searching the medical world for answers to my physical pain. Doctors, specialists, physiotherapists, osteopaths, chiropractors, scans, X-rays, and a myriad of gadgets all provided little relief. This mysterious condition manifested as daily pain in my skull, eyes, neck, shoulders, back, arms, hands, and hips. Some days the pain felt dull and deep, like a familiar ache. Other days its expression was sharp and swift, often catching me off guard and taking my breath away.

There were times when I was positive something in my physical body must be broken, torn, or out of place. Other days, the pain had an emotional element to it, almost as if it was sadness finding a home in my physical body.

During this time, I also had much to celebrate and be grateful for. My three gorgeous boys (then five, six, and eight years old) were happy and healthy. I had a loving husband, a supportive social network, and was in the process of an exciting career reinvention, moving from the not-for-profit sector to the mindfulness and meditation space.

But there were moments when the pain overshadowed all these positives. At times, it felt like there was a sheet of glass between me and the life that I loved and valued. This negative cycle of pain and fear was all pervasive. It took charge of my thoughts, actions, emotions, and at times, my identity.

Globally, it is estimated that one in five, or about 1.5 billion people suffer from chronic pain. For each of these people, their experience will be unique. Chronic pain can be unpredictable and inconsistent. And so was my response to it. Some days, I was fiercely strong and optimistic, and other days I felt tired and defeated. Sometimes I let people in, allowing family and friends to see me in my vulnerability. Other times I pushed people away.

You don't need to have experienced chronic pain to relate to my story or to find comfort in this book. We all have our own personal challenges, whether it's everyday stumbling blocks, an event that has caught us off guard and changed the trajectory of our lives, long-term emotional hurt, or mental health struggles. The lessons I learnt living with chronic pain are universal. You can use them to help you face all kinds of adversity in more skilful ways.

The truth is, nobody's life is perfect, and the sooner we realise that we can be happy, even amidst our challenges, the more empowered we will feel. I have learnt this from personal experience (the hard way!) and by helping people across the world lean into their painful experiences — and really value the fullness of life.

Four years ago, at the age of forty, I was formally diagnosed with fibromyalgia — a chronic pain condition that results in your nervous system getting caught in a state of constant 'wind up'. In other words, my nervous system was *stuck* at a nine out of ten all the time. This was not a relaxing place to be! My brain responded to this permanent state of agitation and arousal by sending signals to my body to produce pain; and the cycle of stress, pain, and fear took hold.

At the time of my diagnosis, I was secretly hoping the doctor would write me a prescription, I'd take a pill, and this chapter in my life would be over. I'd recommence all the activities I loved: playing with my kids, teaching mindfulness, and exercising. I'd reconnect with family and friends. I'd return to the more youthful and vibrant version of me from my past.

But, instead of a prescription, the pain specialist offered me these words: 'There is no pill you can take for this condition. There is also no cure. All you can do is change the way you respond to the pain.'

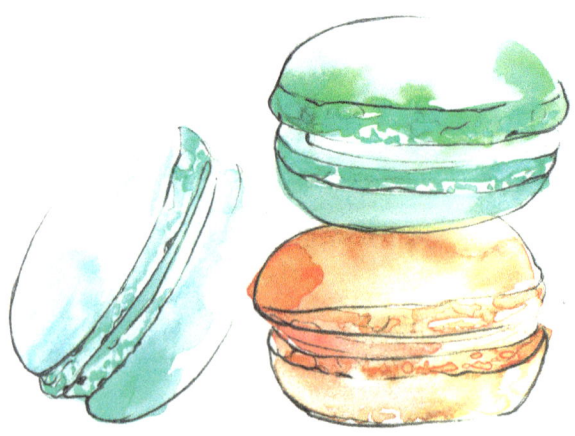

I didn't realise it at the time, but that advice would become my mission. Over the next two years, subconsciously at first and then very consciously, I went on a quest to discover how I could reframe my attitude to pain, both physical and emotional.

My recovery (or healing, if you prefer that word) was, and continues to be, filled with experimentation and humour. There was a stint on medical marijuana which my kids objected to as I ate every sweet thing — or 'special treat' as we call them — in the pantry.

There was past life healing (apparently, I used to be a man and was still carrying the wounds of being left at the altar by the love of my life hundreds of years ago). There were acts of solidarity as my kids and I chanted together in supermarket queues. Did you know, it's almost impossible to sing and feel pain at the same time? (There are plenty more quirky science-backed tips in this book.)

There were changes to my diet and way of life. I embraced a gluten-free lifestyle, became vegetarian, and meditated so frequently it felt more like a spiritual boot camp than relaxation. I even tried juggling to rewire my brain (in case you are wondering, this experiment was unsuccessful).

My all-time favourite was a bizarre car chase between me and my loving mother. Distressed after a doctor's appointment, I had a 'small' breakdown in the car park. My mum tried to calm me down, but instead of allowing her words to soothe me, I jumped in my car and sped off like a middle-aged maniac. She was so concerned, she followed me … and I just couldn't shake this seventy-year-old speedster! When I finally got out of the car and saw her pull up behind me, I laughed and cried at the same time. It was a ridiculous situation, but one that has etched in my mind as a moment of deep healing — a time when I knew that, despite my erratic behaviour, I was not alone.

And then, amidst the special treats and the car chases, there was one very ordinary day that held the deepest healing of all. I was at home (the kids were at school), and I was experiencing a 'pain episode'. The pain wasn't unusual, it travelled its familiar path behind my eyes, down my neck, deep into my shoulders, and down my spine. What was unusual was my response to it.

I wasn't criticising myself for what I might have done to bring it on, nor was I feeling anxious about how long it would stay. Instead, I was being with the pain with curiosity and acceptance. I was noticing the sensations in my body without fear or judgement. I felt strangely calm. And in this radical act of surrender, I was coming home to my deeper nature, to the part of me that was stronger and wiser than the pain. I realised, with clarity, that despite my pain, I was in that moment … happy!

It was not the version of happiness that looks like a happy ending in a nineties rom-com movie. It was a happiness that felt more like a deep experience of presence, connection, and ultimately, peace. The courage to not push anything away, to meet my entire experience in that moment. It felt liberating and exciting. I could sense the relief in my body, mind, and heart. I felt lighter and more free than I'd felt in years.

Suddenly, the doctor's words made sense, 'All you can do is change the way you respond to the pain.' I realised that, as I let go of the resistance, the pain was subsiding. This moment was like a magical seed. Just as the acorn seed contains everything it needs to grow into a powerful oak tree, I knew that this moment held the blueprint for a new way of interacting with life, both the challenges and the joys.

Over the coming months I experimented and reflected. I continued to water this seed with curiosity, creativity, and a quiet determination, until it grew into my 'ten pathways framework': a personally and professionally tested, science-backed and spiritually informed road map for redefining happiness.

Using this framework, I created my app, *The Happy Habit*, and this book, to help people embrace their entire lives — even the parts which caught them by surprise. Over the past three years I've witnessed hundreds of thousands of people around the world explore these pathways as a way of moving beyond life's challenges towards a more vibrant, purposeful, and happy existence.

These pathways may take you out of your comfort zone and ask you to break away from old habits and beliefs. Sometimes change feels both uncomfortable and exciting, and that's okay. If you're here reading this book, you know the *cost* of staying the same, of continuing to resist your challenges whilst 'chasing happiness', is too great.

At first, you may need to consciously work these pathways to make them work for you. This book is here for you whenever you need it. Read it once and then revisit it. Enjoy the beautiful artwork, take a moment to notice how the illustrations make you feel. Come back to your favourite practices. Over time, you'll notice that you don't need to try hard in order to access these pathways. They will be there, like a loyal friend, ready to guide you through the many twists and turns of life.

Finally, if you've never meditated before or you're positive you're not the meditating 'type', rest assured that this is not a meditation book. You won't be asked to sit cross-legged and battle your busy mind, I promise.

We all have pain. It's a shared human experience. My pain was primarily physical. Perhaps your pain includes regret, grief, loss, or loneliness. Maybe your discomfort relates to not feeling lovable or worthy. Whatever your experience, there's a pathway you can explore to feel happier.

As you begin your journey, may you remember that happiness is not the absence of adversity, but the ability to walk alongside these moments and learn from them. As you grow in your capacity to be with the challenges, fears, and scars, may you be rewarded with a bigger, bolder, and more beautiful life.

Ready to do this? Read on ...

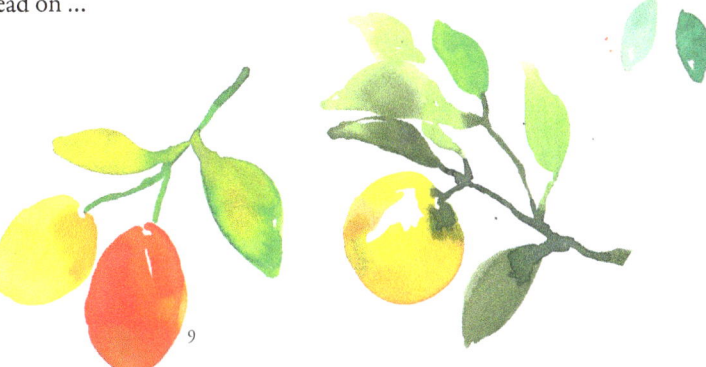

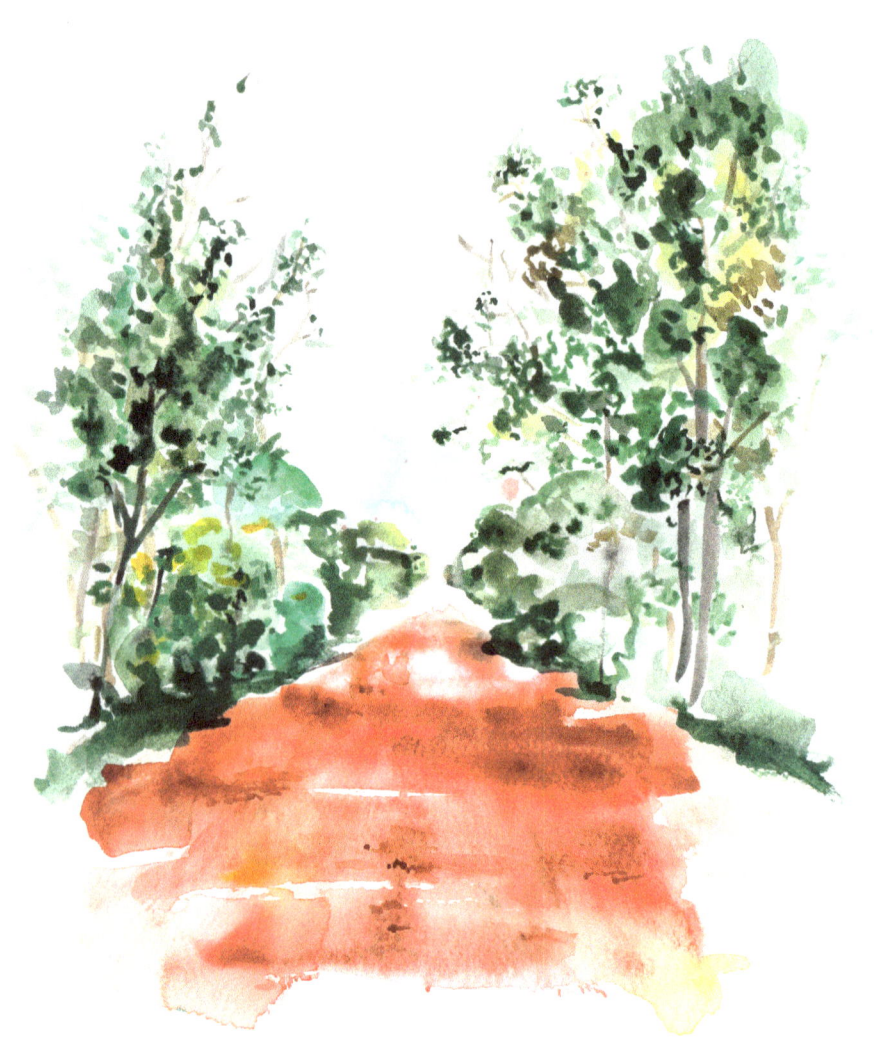

INTRODUCTION

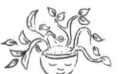

EXERCISE: MEET YOUR TRAVEL COMPANIONS

When we set out on the journey to understand ourselves in new ways and improve our lives, it's important to invite three travel companions: curiosity, courage, and a sense of humour. Think of these qualities or attitudes as friends who will encourage you to keep putting one foot in front of the other even when you are tired, who will pick you up when you fall, and make the trip more enjoyable.

You can welcome these three travel companions now.

It's easy, just close your eyes and take three deep breaths.

Feel your feet on the ground.

Relax your body just a little.

Allow a gentle smile to fall across your lips.

Repeat silently in your mind:

May I be curious.

May I be courageous.

May I smile at my contractions and my funny little ways.

May I accept who I am right now, whilst also holding the intention to transform and grow.

Take a deep breath into these words.

Allow them to land in your mind, body, and heart.

Trust that you are ready.

PATHWAY ONE: AWARENESS

Where attention goes, energy flows

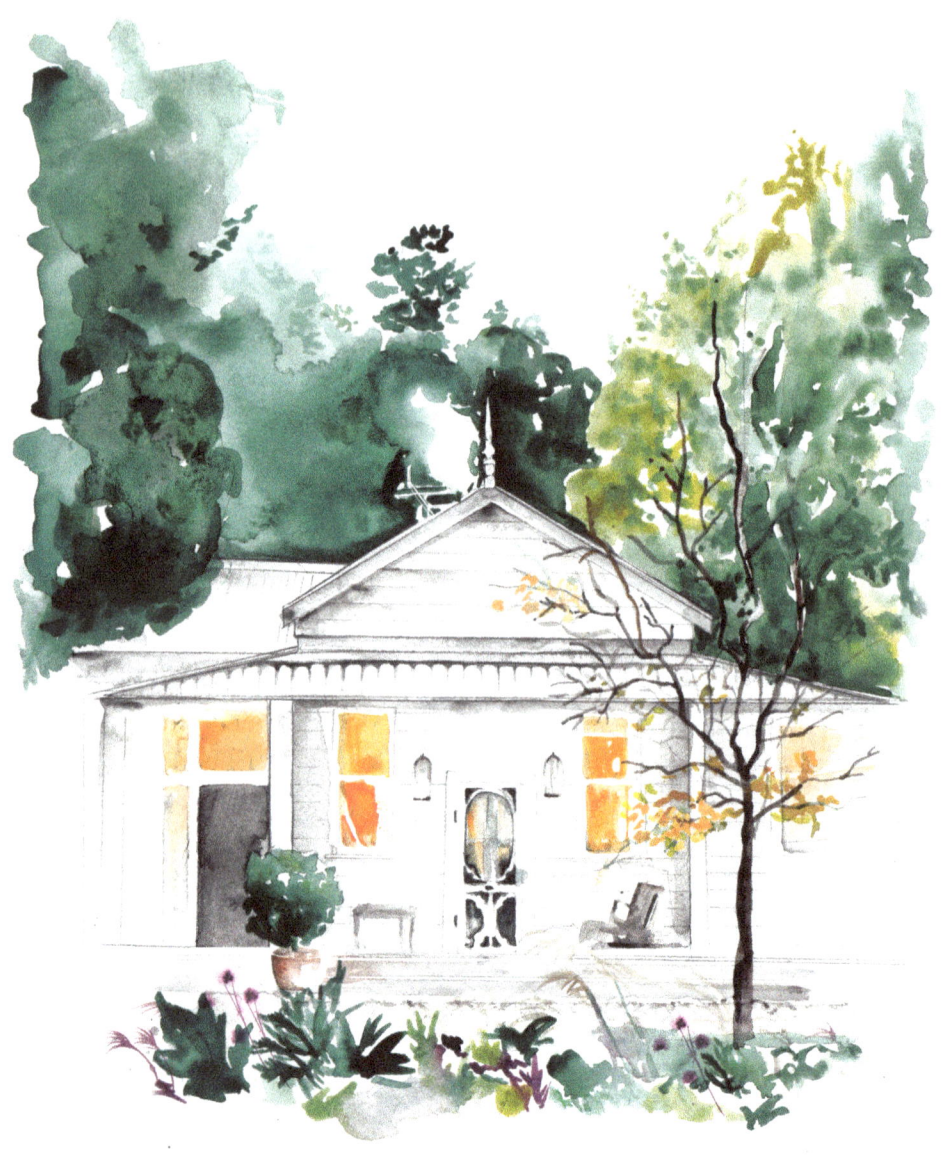

> *You are not your thoughts;*
> *you are the curious and wise*
> *awareness that notices*
> *these thoughts.*

It was a regular Tuesday afternoon in autumn. The sun's rays were gentle, casting shadows across my lawn. I was standing barefoot in my back garden, cool grass nestled between my toes, talking to my mum on the phone. My children (one, two, and four years old), were enjoying filling buckets with soil and water. It was both joyful and messy.

The conversation between my mother and I followed its usual trajectory. I'd share my 'news'. Tom, my eldest son, had brought a painting home from his new kindergarten. Gabe was learning to ride his blue scooter. Dash, my youngest, had decided that bum-shuffling was a better way to keep up with his older brothers than learning to crawl.

My family had just moved across town to a new neighbourhood. It was a beautiful part of the world, but for now, I was yet to establish any real connections.

My mum and I had phoned each other at least once a week for most of my adult life. However, over recent months, there was a new addition to our familiar chats — my tears. Sometimes, the tears would come from sleep deprivation, other times from my mother's kindness and understanding. On this day, the strong flow of emotion stemmed from a conversation I'd just had with a stranger in the park.

This man — another parent — had shared, with great honesty and vulnerability, the fears he held for his child who had a disability. I can't remember how we moved from small talk to such a deep conversation. But at one point, he looked me in the eyes and asked, 'Who will look after my son when I die?' I had no idea what to reply to him. At that moment, I wished I could take his pain away.

As I repeated this story to my mother, warm tears were streaming down my face. I knew, at an intellectual level, that it wasn't my responsibility to provide this distressed stranger with an answer to his question. But his words sat like a 20lb weight on my heart. It felt hard to breathe.

At the time, it felt like everyone, both friends and strangers, had a painful story to share with me. Everywhere I looked there was a real heaviness — and collective sadness. It felt like the autumn breeze carried with it the energy of fear. Each of these interactions would stay with me, like a shadow I couldn't shake. I'd be bathing the kids, reading their bedtime stories, or tidying the house, and these stories would be playing like a record on repeat in my mind.

As I write this, Australia (and the entire world) is coming out of a turbulent period of lockdowns, restrictions, and pandemic living. Fear and uncertainty have certainly been the pervasive culture over the last two years. I know many of you will relate to this feeling of being surrounded by stories that pull at your heartstrings and make you feel both helpless and unsettled.

Ever since I was a child, I've been extremely compassionate. When I was eight years old, I would say a little prayer each time I heard the siren of an ambulance, sending my best wishes to whoever was on their way to hospital (I'll get to the significance of our childhood more in other chapters).

I spent much of my twenties working at a large not-for-profit organisation providing support for people experiencing disadvantage, including disability. During this time, I was surrounded by examples of how life could be hard, unfair, and painful for people. But I also felt hopeful and able to see the joy in the world too.

I have always been ready and willing to 'offer a shoulder to cry on', someone who people naturally confide in. What had changed in recent times was my response to the stories that people were sharing with me. It was beginning to feel uncalibrated and too much to handle. I felt like a tree without roots, being blown about by the wind and the rain that was other people's lives, engulfed in a cloud of generalised fear and heaviness.

I found myself shifting into victim mode: *Why does everyone always tell their sad stories to me?* I felt like a magnet for pain, sadness, disappointment, and regret, and I didn't know how much more I could process.

This combination of compassion and resentment made me feel both uneasy and guilty. It certainly wasn't helping with the day-to-day reality of parenting three very small children.

My mum, who knows me better than anyone, had noticed the heightened sensitivity that was growing within me. During this phone call, she seized her moment and said to me in a firm but loving voice, 'Darl, you really need to start practicing mindfulness, so you can feel stronger for yourself and those three gorgeous kids of yours.'

Growing up, Mum was a psychologist who, to her credit, refrained from 'putting me on the therapist's couch' too often. Over the years she had suggested I try mindfulness, but this time her words landed in a different way. I felt desperate.

Maybe this would be the answer. So began my journey into mindfulness and meditation.

Eleven years later, I look back at that version of myself — the young and tired mother — and I notice three interrelated things:

1. **My self-imposed high expectations.** My desire to be a perfect mother and my desperate attempts to control life had created stress within my body, distraction within my mind, and a heaviness within my heart.

2. **My negative perspective.** Over time, living this way was like putting on a pair of sunglasses with lenses that were tinted with fear and scarcity. The longer I wore these glasses, the more sad stories I would see and hear, until my perspective of the world became skewed towards the negative. As each day passed, a growing belief that the world was not a safe place sank deep into my bones. And so, the cycle of control and fear continued.

3. **I was desperately lonely.** Yes, lonely! A strange thing to consider given I was never alone. In fact, during that period in my life there was always a little person on my hip or at my side, even when I went to the bathroom. I now know that this loneliness was a call home to my deeper nature. It was an invitation back into my body, my heart, and an abiding sense that the world, despite its challenges, was a safe place. It was a gentle whisper to loosen my grip and instead begin to trust life.

Over the years, my mindfulness and meditation practices have transformed and grown just as I have. Sometimes, it does look very formal (repeating mantras whilst sitting cross-legged on the floor). Other times it looks more like 'beditation', the practice of meditating whilst all warm and cosy in my bed.

There's been sound healing, chanting, energy work, and psychotherapy. Even dance has played its part. I've dived deep into the pool of my emotions and limiting beliefs. I've also explored the mind-body connection (more on that later).

I've found healing in nature, compassion, love, and letting go. Along the way some practices have become like old and loyal friends, ready to support me whatever my circumstance. They've helped me reorientate my awareness away from fear towards greater presence and peace. May they support you as you walk the pathway of awareness.

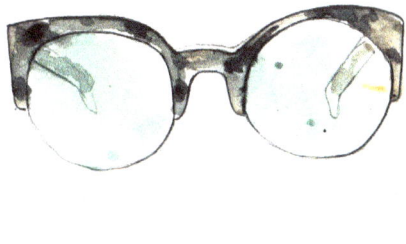

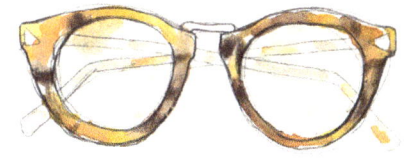

WHILST THE WORD 'SAFE' DOESN'T FEEL VERY EXCITING OR SEXY, OUR NERVOUS SYSTEM LOVES IT!

Safety: fake it till you feel it

Whilst the word 'safe' doesn't feel very exciting or sexy, our nervous system loves it! When our command centre feels safe, the positive flow-on effects are far reaching. When our bodies feel safe our immune and digestive systems work more effectively, we are more able to heal and regenerate at a cellular level. When our reptilian brain feels safe, we can think clearly, broaden our perspective, and creatively problem-solve. When our hearts feel safe we can navigate our emotions more skilfully, communicate our needs more honestly, and forgive others and ourselves.

Life feels easier when we get in the habit of pausing and reminding ourselves that we are safe. We are more able to recover from stress, illness and injury, to bounce back from everyday setbacks, to acknowledge the opinions and perspectives of others, and to maintain healthy relationships.

So, how can we send ourselves a message that we are safe? It starts with simple steps to soothe yourself. For me, this included sitting barefoot in my backyard and feeling my feet in the cool grass. Becoming more open about my fears and worries with my family and support network. Reminding myself that mistakes are a natural part of being a parent. And my all-time favourite, really acknowledging how all my children were tucked up in bed, safe and sound, before I drifted off to sleep.

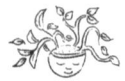

EXERCISE: A SAFETY RESET

Find a quiet place to sit at home, maybe on your bed or in the living room.

Begin by simply casting your eye around the space you are in, really noticing the basic features of your environment that provide you with a sense of safety. Perhaps you notice the door, its handle, the windows, the way they open and close, or the roof over your head.

Move your awareness to some of the aspects of your room that allow you to feel comfortable and at home. Maybe there's a photo or picture, an indoor plant, a book, or your favourite blanket or jumper. Perhaps the way the sunlight streams in makes you feel relaxed and at ease.

Remind yourself that this space doesn't need to be perfect or even tidy in order to offer you a feeling of safety.

Take a few deep breaths into this moment, really imagining this experience of being safe landing within your body, mind, and heart.

Notice any changes in your physical body. Notice any changes in your emotional world.

Repeat silently in your mind:

Right here, right now, I am safe, I am free from harm.

Offer this moment of awareness a smile! You've just recalibrated your nervous system. Trust that this safety reset will create positive ripples in your day.

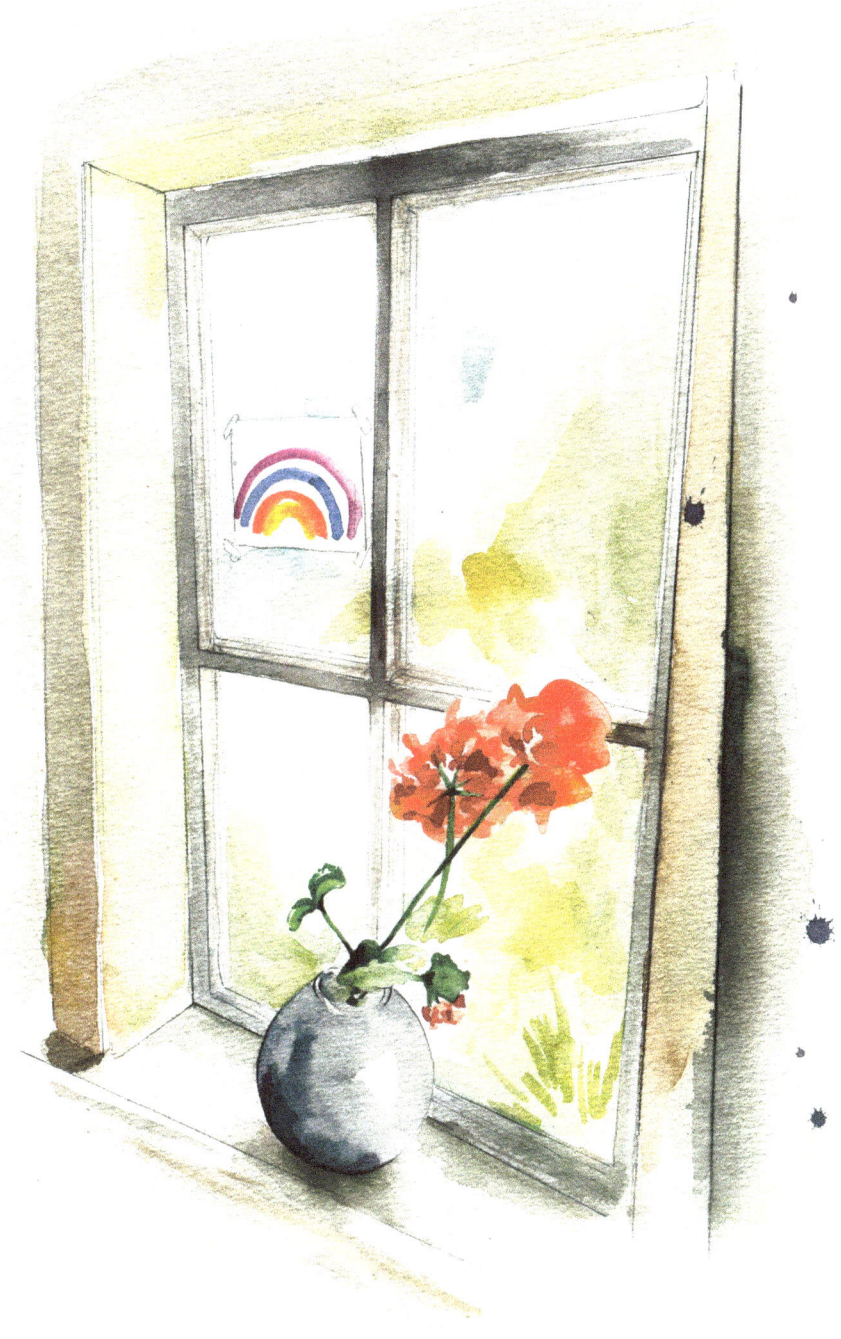

Doing this practice once a day all those years ago allowed me to take off those glasses that were tinted with fear. Amazingly, when I did, I was more able to respond to life's challenges, both other people's and my own, with a relaxed body, a clear head, and a wise and open heart.

The dangers of distraction

Sometimes it feels like everyone, and everything, is vying for a slice of our attention. Our phones, computers, and other devices are luring us in with their incessant dinging. Work requires more and more from us each day. Even our family and friends are wanting our time.

Our busy minds add to this distraction. Whilst eating breakfast or having our morning coffee or tea, we are frequently lost in thought, planning and rehearsing the day ahead, often with a quiet feeling of dread or worry about how we will fit it all in. Whilst exercising or taking a walk, we replay conversations and situations over and over, wishing things had played out differently. We lie in bed at night being hard on ourselves or judging others.

Research conducted by Harvard psychologists, Matthew Killingsworth and Daniel Gilbert, estimates that humans spend 47% of our waking hours thinking about something other than our immediate environment. In their article, 'A wandering mind is an unhappy mind', they highlight the dangers of this level of distraction, stating, 'How often our minds leave the present and where they tend to go is a better predictor of our happiness than the activities in which we are engaged.'

Research confirms what Eastern traditions, Western science, and our own hearts have been telling us all along — happiness is to be found in the present moment and has more to do with our attention and less to do with the situation itself.

As crazy as it sounds, you could experience a deeper level of happiness whilst mindfully preparing a meal than by laying on a beautiful beach thinking about all the things you need to do when you get home or how wobbly your thighs are.

An important aspect of walking towards a new version of happiness is reminding yourself each day that you get to *choose* where you place your attention. You get to choose what stories, ideas, and drama you focus on, and what you let go. At times, swimming against the tide of distraction can feel hard, but it's worth it. As they say in Tibetan culture, take care of the minutes and the years will take care of themselves.

We can begin to break free from this trance of mental distraction by really using all our senses.

Sight

In every moment, our eyes are taking in colours, shapes, textures, the faces of those we love, and clouds as they cross the sky.

Sound

Our ears are allowing us to connect with the world more fully, offering us the gift of conversation, music, and laughter.

Taste

We receive the pleasure of tasting a perfect piece of summer fruit, a slice of cake, or a delicious home-cooked meal.

Smell

We experience a gentle rush of delight as we smell flowers in bloom, our morning coffee, or fresh bread from the bakery.

Touch

We feel the cool air greet our skin on a winter's morning or the warm sand beneath our feet on a summer's day.

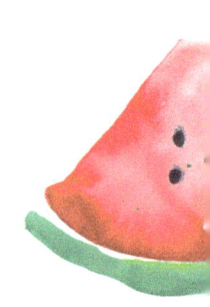

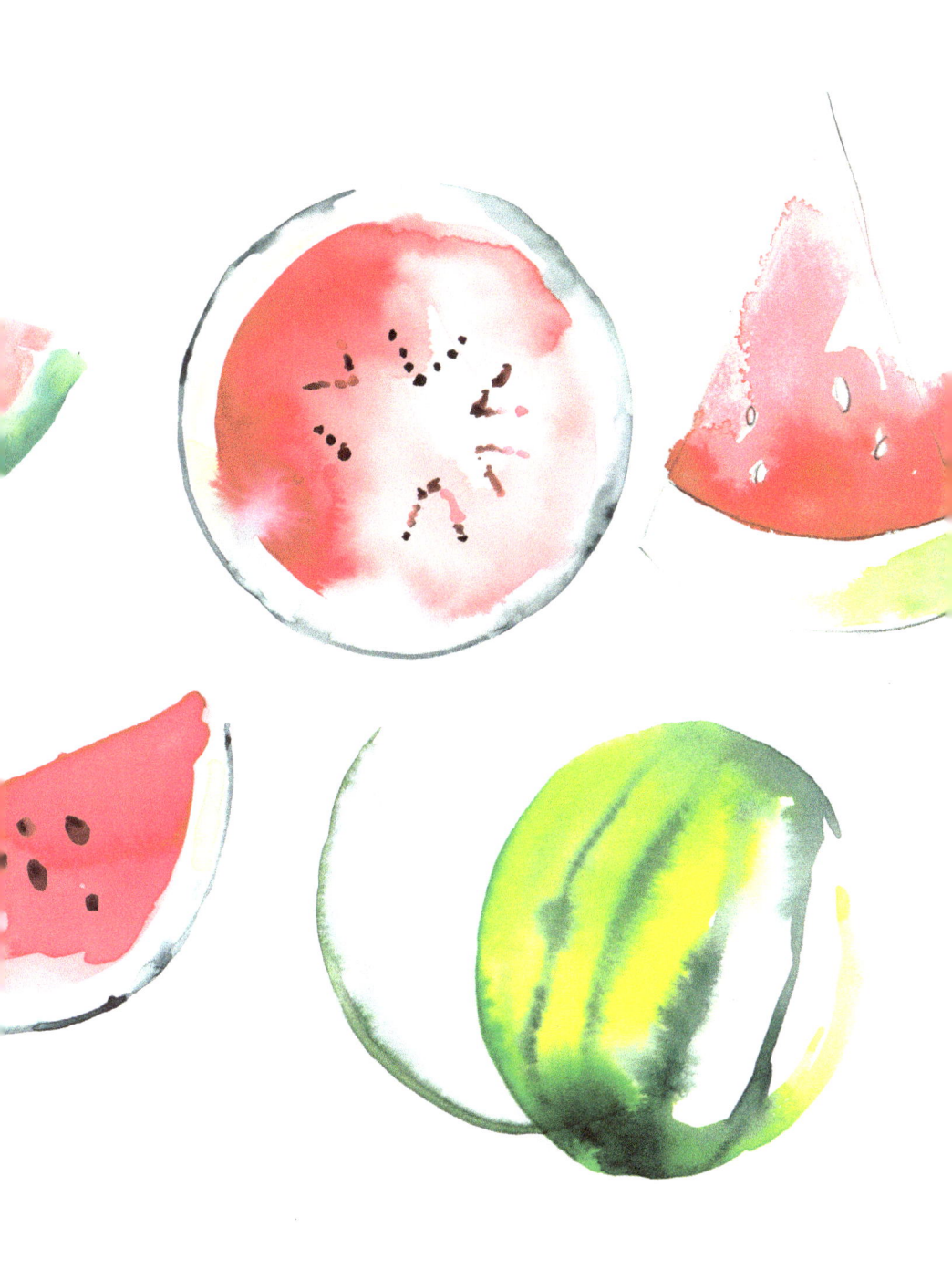

Taking the time each day to be in your sensate world is a simple yet powerful practice that will help you come down from your busy mind into the fullness of the present moment — the place where happiness resides.

The difference between thinking and sensing

During my meditation teacher training I learnt a simple fact that changed my life: it's not possible to *think* and *sense* at the same time. This is because thinking results in fast, erratic 'beta' brain waves, whilst sensing produces the slower, more rhythmic 'alpha' brain waves. Generally speaking, thinking arouses you, whilst sensing serves to relax you. Sensing also offers the bonus of a well-deserved break from all that rumination, planning, judgement, self-criticism, or worry.

With so much pleasure to experience through our senses, and with the tendency for our minds to focus on the negative, it seems both strange and sad that we spend so little time here — in the sensing space. I guess advertisers wouldn't profit from promoting this way of life as it doesn't require us to make a purchase or an upgrade.

Now that you are aware of the difference between the thinking and sensing modes, I hope you'll explore the world of sight, sound, taste, smell, and touch more. You'll be surprised how quickly you notice a change within you.

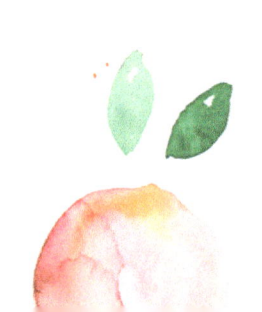

EXERCISE: ACTIVATE YOUR SENSES

Begin by taking one deep breath. Notice the temperature of the air as it enters your body. Notice the sound of the air as it leaves your body.

Feel the parts of your body that meet the ground beneath you. Focus on this point of connection for a moment.

Notice sounds in your immediate environment. Notice sounds far away. Notice sounds close by. Pick up on the moments of silence between the sounds.

Take in the details of your immediate environment. Notice (as if for the first time) the different shapes, colours, and textures. Can you see something with fresh eyes?

Take another deep breath. Notice how your whole body expands as you breath in, and your whole body contracts as you breath out.

Soften the space above your eyes, your shoulders, your belly.

Enjoy three life-affirming breaths as you remember that you are a full sensing body, not just a mind.

Repeat after me: You are not your thoughts.

With over 60,000 thoughts per day, it's no wonder so many of us live primarily in our heads. Given that so many of our thoughts have a negative, cautionary tone to them, and they take us away from the present moment, it's wise to develop a more discerning relationship with our thoughts. This doesn't require expensive therapy or a calm and still mind; you can start by asking this simple question:

> Where are my thoughts taking me right now?

Perhaps they've transported you back in time, to a particular conversation or situation. Maybe they've allowed you to time travel into the future, as you imagine all the things you need to do tomorrow, or you fantasise about the weekend.

From here, you can get curious and ask yourself:

> If this thought had a name, what would I call it?

Some common thinking habits include ruminating, replaying, regretting, worrying, planning, strategising, rehearsing, hoping, wishing, and wanting.

Notice also if these thinking habits contain words or phrases like:

> If only I/they
> I can't believe I/they
> I should
> I need to
> I wish

Well done. By answering these two questions you've already broken free from whatever thinking trance you were caught in. This simple practice has created space between you and your thoughts. This space is your ticket to freedom and happiness.

You can deepen this practice by asking your thoughts three more questions:

1. Are you kind?
2. Do you help me be the person I want to be?
3. How do you make me feel about myself or my life?

There's no right or wrong answer to these questions. They are designed to circuit-break the trance-like quality of your thoughts and the feeling of being pulled in by them. These questions also allow you to see that you are not your thoughts, you are the curious and wise awareness that notices these thoughts.

From here, you'll be more able to shift into sensing mode and enjoy the pleasure and safety found in the present moment. Cherish your awareness as you would a small child. I hope you'll have the courage to gently guide it home to the truth of what really matters each time it loses its way.

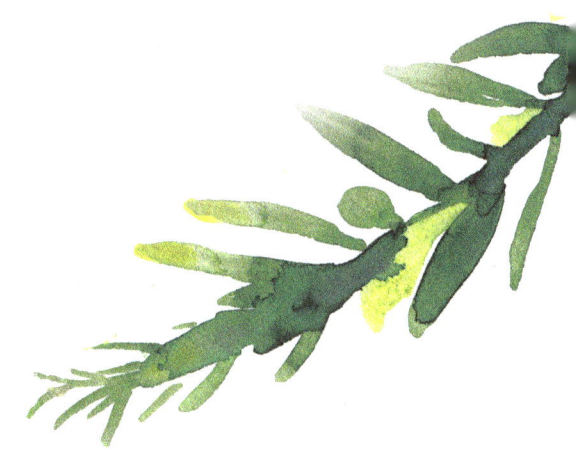

PATHWAY TWO: COMPASSION

The first and second arrows

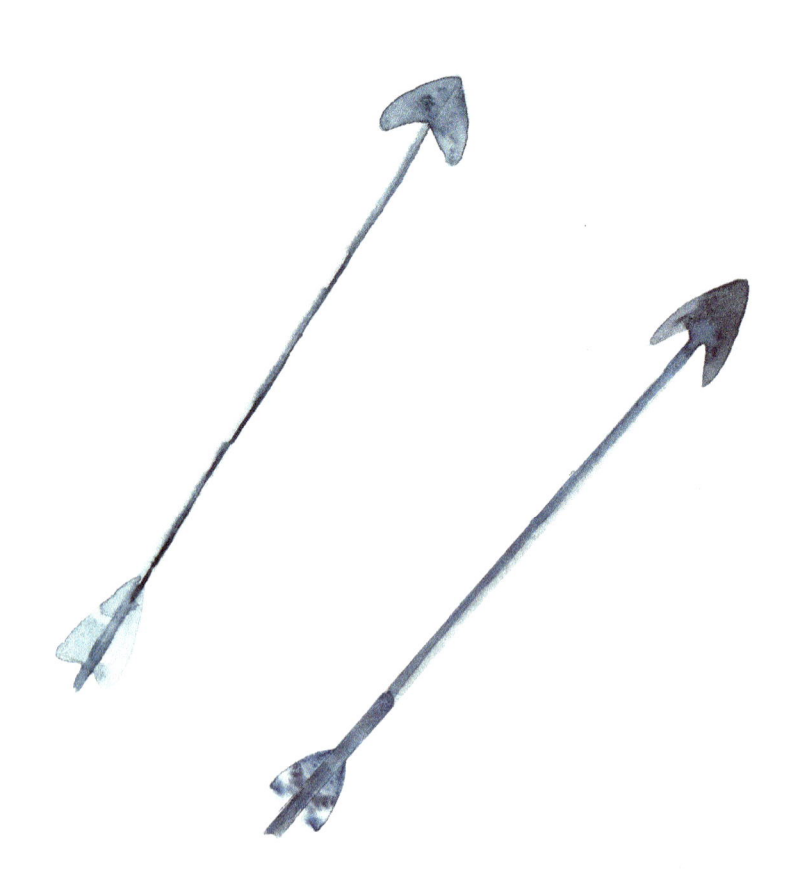

Are my expectations causing this suffering? What story or meaning have I attached to this moment?

When challenges come our way — whether in our relationships, at work or within our emotional, mental, or physical world — a tsunami of emotion often trails in the wake. The guilt that swells after separation, the shame that washes in during a period of heightened anxiety or the self-judgement that rises to the surface after job loss or illness. Often these experiences cause us more harm than the initial situation itself.

This idea of first and second waves of pain and suffering has its origins in Buddhist philosophy. In his teaching of the Sallatha Sutta (translated to 'the arrow'), the Buddha explains that suffering is like being shot by two arrows:

> **First arrow:** The initial pain caused by the primary event or circumstance. We will all experience these arrows in our lifetime, it's a natural part of the human experience.

> **Second arrow:** The mental and emotional suffering that arises as we assign meaning to the first arrow. It includes, for example, all the 'why me' or 'poor me' narratives we tell ourselves and the 'it's my fault' or 'I deserved this' stories. The second arrow also includes the feelings of shame, regret, remorse, inner judgement, and loneliness that often accompany the moments of stress in our lives.

Often these stories — the second arrows — hurt for longer than the initial complaint. They can even have a negative impact on our identity long after the first wave of pain has passed. After one relationship break-up, we take on the identity of being unlovable. After a work restructure resulting in a period of job loss, we see ourselves as permanently unemployable.

Looking back to the time of my formal fibromyalgia diagnosis, I can see clearly how the second arrows of suffering began almost immediately. A rush of shame washed over me as soon as I heard the doctor's words, 'There is no pill you can take for this condition. There is also no cure. All you can do is change the way you respond to the pain.'

At that moment, all I heard was, 'You are foolish for thinking there would be a pill for your condition. You aren't coping well enough with the pain. You should be managing your situation better.'

His words pulled at the frays of my identity. They challenged a core belief I held about myself that I was strong, good at coping, and rarely reliant on others for help. Given that this identity had roots that travelled deep into the earth of my childhood — and served the important function of helping me to feel safe — it's no surprise that I suffered when this belief was called into question. So, there I was, sitting in the doctor's office, feeling like someone had pulled a rug of safety from beneath my physical and emotional bodies.

Over the following months, there were many more triggering interactions that lead to a second layer of pain and suffering. Several well-meaning friends tried to offer me support by saying, 'There's no way you have fibromyalgia — that's only for people who have experienced *real* trauma in their past, and you had a great childhood.' Instead of soothing me, these words sparked an uncomfortable inner dialogue that I was both privileged and weak.

I was left wondering: *How could I have a condition that is reserved for people who have lived through significant stress or trauma in their lives?* Hello, second arrows of guilt and shame.

When the neurologist looked over the results of my brain scan, he said to me, 'Wow, you are really stressed for a meditation teacher!' That arrow hit hard, as it made me question my professional authenticity. I felt like an imposter in the wellness industry, the equivalent of a naturopath who secretly gorged on McDonald's or the family therapist who hadn't spoken to her teenage kids for months. Having a nervous system that was locked in a state of perpetual stress was bad enough. Adding these second arrows resulted in a new level of inner pain and turmoil.

With the passage of time, I can see that all these people meant no harm. I understand that my response to their comments owed more to my frazzled nervous system than to their actual words or intentions. But here's another aspect of living with chronic pain and a revved-up command centre that no-one talks about: everything feels like a threat or a criticism. According to my reptilian brain, I was surrounded by lions prowling in the distance.

My experience of heightened sensitivity towards the comments of others during a period of stress isn't unique. Nor were the feelings of guilt, shame, and inner judgement that rolled in as I navigated my health challenge. This hypersensitivity and swell of uncalibrated emotions is a common side effect of stress and something that many of us experience when navigating challenges in our lives. At a time when we could really benefit from connection and support, we end up feeling judged and alone.

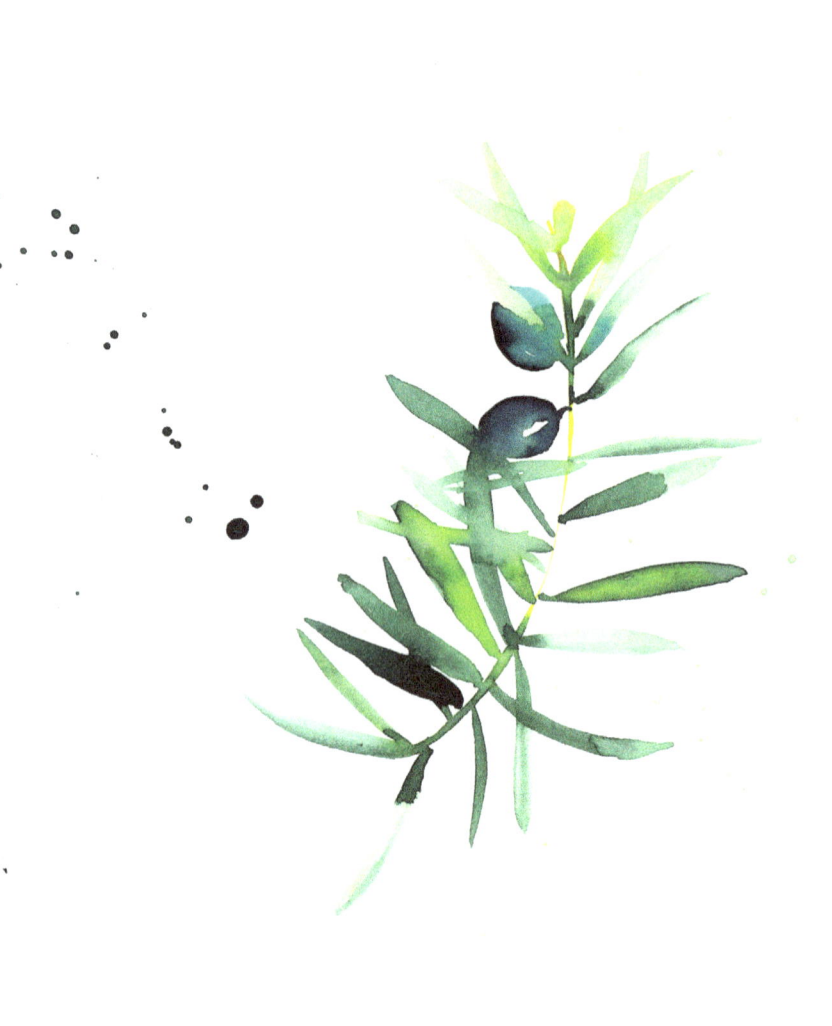

EXERCISE: YOUR SECOND ARROWS

Pause and take three deep breaths.

Think back to a difficult time in your life — whatever first springs to mind.

Try as best you can to describe the first arrow (the primary event or situation).

Now explore your second arrows by reflecting on these two questions:

What emotions did you experience as a result of this challenging time and how did they make you feel about yourself and your identity?

Did you have any interactions with others that increased your pain or suffering?

Breathe deeply and repeat silently in your mind:

I offer these second arrows, and myself, compassion.

Well done. It takes courage to differentiate between the first and second waves of pain and suffering. But each time we do this, we are more able to alter our response, and ultimately, protect ourselves.

In order to heal, we need to feel

My journey towards greater health and a new definition of happiness consisted of more time exploring these second arrows than the first arrow — that being the physical pain itself. During the months after my diagnosis, whenever I experienced pain, felt triggered, or noticed strong emotions, I asked myself this simple question:

Is this a first or second arrow experience?

If I identified it as a first arrow experience, I offered it, and myself, compassion. I did this by breathing deeply and noticing physical sensations and emotions. I tried my best not to push anything away, to just be with what was there. I offered myself clear and supportive phrases like *Life feels really hard right now*, and *It's okay to feel this way*.

I reminded myself that even though it felt uncomfortable, this moment was good for me. I gently encouraged my body to soften and feel at ease. Really feeling the pain of the first arrow and offering it compassion is a crucial step in healing. When we do this, we reduce the number of second arrows that come our way.

With so much talk about compassion in books and on social media, it's easy to feel overwhelmed or worried you aren't doing it correctly. In truth, there's no right or wrong way to offer yourself compassion. It's more about just being with your experience and allowing felt sensations and emotions to come and go without burying or resisting them. It also includes reminding yourself that we all have hard times and that the rough patches are just a natural part of being human.

So, what about those second arrows? If I noticed that what I was navigating felt more like a second arrow (the story or meaning I was assigning to the situation), the first step was the same — compassion. So, how could I be more kind to myself?

Again, I slowed down my breath. I noticed physical sensations and emotions come and go. The next step was curiosity. I reminded myself of the Buddha's teachings, that we can reduce the severity of the second arrow through our wise attention and intention. I asked myself these questions as a way of understanding my experience more:

- Are my expectations causing this suffering?
- If I soften the expectations I have of myself, others, or the way life 'should' be, does the suffering subside?
- What story or meaning have I assigned to this moment? Is this interpretation a help or a hindrance to my wellbeing?
- What is the real pain of this situation?
- How can I offer this first arrow my compassion?

I also took my compassion one step further. I asked myself: *Is there another person I could offer compassion to?* Often our second arrow is caused by someone saying something that triggers us (like my doctor or my well-meaning friends). If so, I would repeat this phrase silently in my mind: *I know you meant no harm. I wish you well.*

Whenever life feels hard or you feel really pulled in by certain situations or conversations, you can ask yourself these same questions. As we discussed in the awareness pathway (revisit it, if you need to), it's not about having the 'right' answer. It's about using curiosity (and compassion) to break the trance-like quality of your thoughts.

Walking towards a new version of happiness is about creating space, and ultimately, freedom. Imagine this space is like a perfect patch of warm grass to sit for a few minutes before you continue along your way. A place to rest your feet and to feel the sun on your face. Because we all know the journey feels easier and more enjoyable after we've taken a little break.

When we dare to meet our pain with warm-hearted awareness, we unlock hidden opportunities. I am grateful for the opportunity to distinguish between the first and second arrows of suffering as this has allowed me to feel more compassionate and less alone. It's also a skill I can use in so many other areas of my life — at work, in my relationships, and at home.

Why it can feel so hard to be kind to ourselves

Of all the ten happiness pathways, compassion is the one that elicits the most resistance and fear in a lot of people I work with. It's also the avenue that is most misunderstood (in close second place is acceptance, but we'll get to that at the end of the book).

In my professional life, I've been fortunate enough to connect with people all around the world. I've received thousands of questions relating to happiness. By far the most common questions relate to self-compassion. People from all different backgrounds and life circumstances ask a version of the same question:

> Will self-compassion make me unmotivated/soft/weak/self-indulgent/lazy?
> The short answer is no.

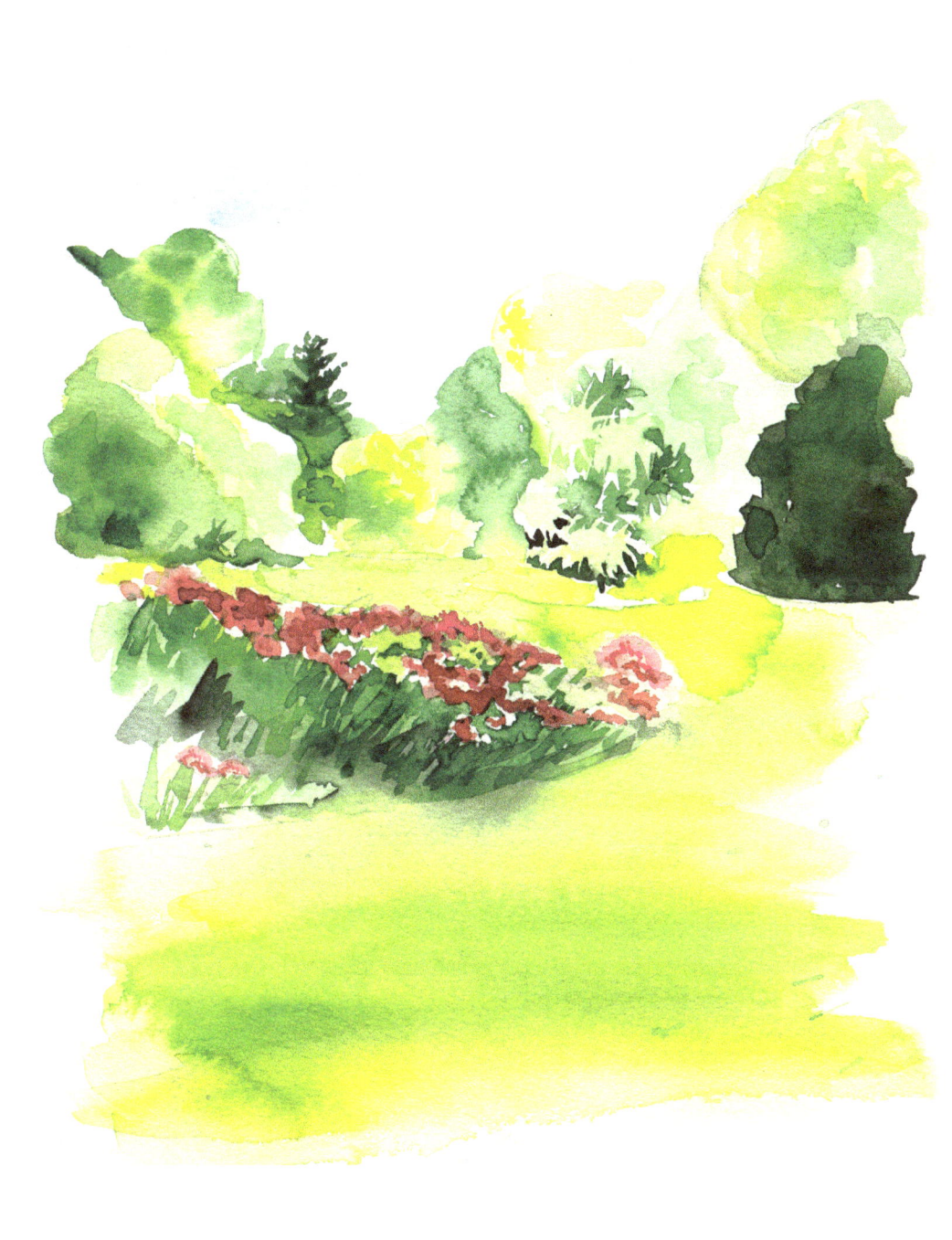

Self-compassion is simply the practice of turning understanding, acceptance, and love inwards. It's about treating yourself in the same way you would treat a good friend. Self-compassion won't strip you of your drive. It won't make you lose your edge. You won't have a pity party for one or turn into a self-centered, unreliable, sleep-until-noon version of yourself.

But self-compassion *might* make you uncomfortable. Many of us have spent a lifetime being hard on ourselves when we don't reach those self-imposed high standards. We've had years of listening to (and believing) the inner dialogue that 'we should have achieved more or been better'. So it's no surprise that starting a more supportive conversation with ourselves can feel unnatural, or even forced, to begin with.

When we shift our inner dynamic towards greater self-friendliness, it can also be shocking to realise just how mean we have been to ourselves over the years. I've certainly had moments, sitting on my bathroom floor, tears streaming down my cheeks, filled with a dual sense of tenderness and remorse. Sitting with the part of you who is deeply loving and kind whilst also acknowledging your inner mean girl is a confronting experience! But I would prefer to move through this shock and uncomfortableness than spend a lifetime in a haze of unfriendliness towards myself. Wouldn't you?

There are thousands of pieces of research highlighting the benefits of practicing self-compassion. In my mind, the most interesting and affirming list comes from Dr Kirsten Neff, the pioneer of self-compassion research. In her books and research papers she articulates beautifully the diverse benefits we receive from this practice.

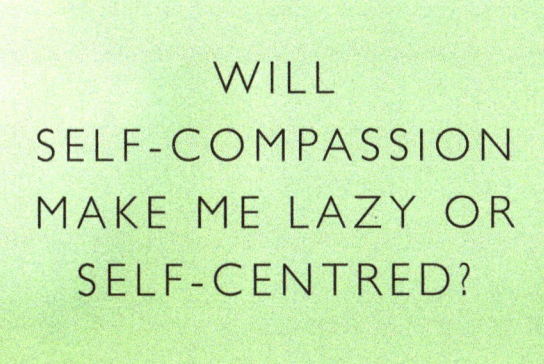

WILL SELF-COMPASSION MAKE ME LAZY OR SELF-CENTRED?

According to Dr Neff, people who practice self-compassion are more able to:

- Cope with tough situations like divorce, trauma, or chronic pain.
- Feel optimistic about their future.
- Buffer themselves from depression, anxiety, and stress.
- Feel resilient and courageous during times of challenge.
- Maintain healthy behaviours like exercising, eating well, drinking less, and going to the doctor more regularly.
- Take personal responsibility for their actions and apologise if they have offended someone.
- Feel motivated to reach their goals.
- Acknowledge that imperfection is part of the human experience.
- Feel into the idea of shared humanity and foster more positive relationships with others.
- Forgive themselves when they don't get things right and move on.
- Cultivate a friendly inner dialogue.

WHEN WE SHIFT OUR INNER DYNAMIC TOWARDS GREATER SELF-FRIENDLINESS, IT CAN BE 'SHOCKING' TO REALISE JUST HOW MEAN WE HAVE BEEN TO OURSELVES OVER THE YEARS.

Given that much of our inner criticism begins within our minds, an important aspect of compassion is creating an inner library of soothing and supportive phrases. When we have these at hand, ready to go, we can respond promptly to the familiar voice of inner doubt, criticism, or judgement before it alters the physiological state of our body. (Yes, negative thoughts create real stress in our bodies.)

Here's a snapshot of my list as inspiration:

Inner Critic	*Inner Ally*
I should have been more patient; I wish I didn't raise my voice.	You've got a lot going on right now, it's okay to apologise and then move on.
I planned on getting more done today, I wish I didn't get so sidetracked.	Life happens. We can't control it. Sometimes we don't get to everything on our to-do list and that's okay. There's always tomorrow.
I wish the house was tidier when my friends came over for dinner.	It's okay for people to see my house when it's messy. People love knowing that I'm not perfect, it makes them feel more relaxed.
I've been eating badly lately.	It's okay to have a piece of cake every now and then. Anyway, it was delicious!

EXERCISE: THE INNER ALLY LIBRARY

Remember that self-compassion is about responding to yourself as you would respond to a friend. As you complete the following exercise, it might help to imagine a friend making these self-critical comments and you responding in supportive ways.

The key to growing your own 'inner ally library' is to develop phrases that feel real to you. Use your own language, not words you think you 'should' use or words you've heard someone else use, which don't feel right to you.

Grab a pen and paper and put two headings across the top of the page: Inner Critic and Inner Ally.

Begin by writing down all the self-critical thoughts or phrases that you often say to yourself. Include the harsh judgements you make, the mean voice. You are aiming for at least seven in this column.

Take a breath. Read over the list and notice how it makes you feel.

Now respond to each of these negative comments with a phrase that feels more supportive, encouraging, or friendly.

Read over these Inner Ally phrases and commit to using them in your everyday life.

If you need a prompt, write them on a Post-it Note, create a screensaver for your laptop or phone, or email it to yourself. Let these act like a pep talk, a reminder that you are safe, you are loved, you matter.

Given that human connection is often cited as one of the key determinants in human happiness, it's also wise to practice softening the judgements we make about friends, family, colleagues, and even strangers so that we can feel closer to the people in our lives.

Here's a snapshot of my list as inspiration:

Outer Judgements	*Outer Friendliness*
I can't believe they said that. Didn't they know that would make me feel ...	They meant no harm.
They always talk about themselves. They are never interested in how I am.	I can see that this person has a lot going on. It felt good to support them. Next time, I'll just offer up my news instead of waiting for them to ask. I'm sure they will be interested.
What they said was hurtful and inconsiderate.	Not everything is about me. We are all trying our best each day. I'm going to choose to not take it so personally.

EXERCISE: THE OUTER FRIENDLINESS LIBRARY

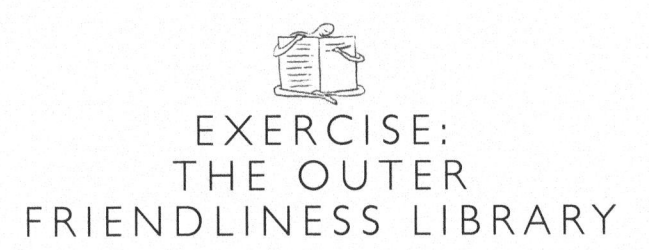

Grab a pen and paper and put two headings across the top of the page: Outer Judgements and Outer Friendliness.

Begin by writing down all the things you say about other people that don't feel particularly kind, true, or necessary.

Take a breath. Read over the list (without getting pulled into the stories or the drama). Let's not judge the judgement!

Now respond to each of these negative comments with a phrase that feels more understanding, generous, and compassionate.

Offer yourself a smile, you've just taken a huge step forward along the pathway of compassion.

Self-compassion — a daily practice, not a last resort

When people come to the practice of self-compassion, it's often from a place of overwhelm, stress, or 'last resort'. I hear it all the time, phrases like 'I really *need* to be more self-compassionate'. It's like people are exhausted from a long trek carrying a backpack full of heavy self-judgement, inner criticism, fear, and blame. They arrive at the end of their journey, tired and desperate, like they couldn't muster another step.

The challenge with arriving at self-compassion from an overwhelmed state or a nervous system on edge is that we often bring our mental stress into the practice. We try self-compassion but our already loud inner critic chimes in, saying things like, *You don't deserve this compassion,* or, *This is silly, it won't work.*

For self-compassion to 'work', we need to arrive at it from our hearts not our minds (and preferably not from an exhausted state). Again, this may feel uncomfortable if you're accustomed to living primarily in your head or if your identity is tied up with being logical, rational, or a good thinker. It may also require you to soften the stories and judgements you have about the heart and people who are 'heart-centred'. Sadly, many of us have been brought up in societies (and families) that applaud toughness, hiding your emotions, and achieving over feeling.

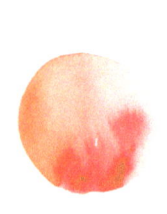

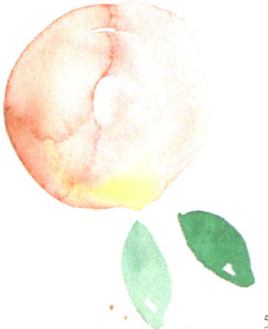

Your stories may sound like:

- The heart is soft, irrational, and full of emotions I can't control.
- My mind is more reliable/honest/trustworthy than my heart.
- I'll have to talk about/express my emotions if I connect with my heart.
- I just don't want to go there, it feels too unfamiliar, heavy, or sad.
- People who are heart-centred are spiritual or 'woo-woo' (and that's not me!).
- People who are heart-centred don't think things through, are irrational, or impulsive.
- If I live from the heart, I'll never be successful or achieve everything I dream of.

When you begin to explore your heart, it's helpful to embrace the attitude of 'beginner's mind'. In Buddhism this concept is known as Shoshin. It relates to having an attitude of openness and a lack of preconceptions when studying a subject. The first line of Zen Master Shunryu Suzuki's seminal book, *Zen Mind, Beginner's Mind,* sums it up powerfully: 'In the beginner's mind there are many possibilities, but in the expert's mind there are a few.'

Over the years I have enjoyed exploring my heart with this beginner's mind. This is what I've discovered.

Your heart will beat about 100,000 times today, 35 million times this year, and over 2 billion times in an average lifetime. All day, every day, it pumps blood with vital nutrients around your body. In one day, your heart helps blood travel up to 19,000km across your body. Over a lifetime, the heart will pump one million barrels of blood. Take a moment to think about this. It's incredible. Don't tell me this isn't a high-achieving organ!

Sir Tom Moore, who, at one hundred years of age, was knighted by Queen

Elizabeth for raising £30 million to support the health care workers during the COVID-19 pandemic, paints the perfect picture in his book, *Captain Tom's Life*:

> *'Every morning, as I open my century-old eyes to another day of life, I lie in bed and allow my body to catch up with my mind. Lying very still, I can feel my heart pounding inside its bony chassis. It's a miracle to me that this old fuel pump has been ticking over since 1920. Thanks to its unfaltering perseverance, yet another day has dawned that I've never seen before. It is certainly one that I will never see again. This fact, alone, is enough to confirm to me that today will be a good day.'*

Research conducted by the HeartMath Institute shows the human heart is more than an effective pump that sustains life. In their book, *Science of the Heart*, the Institute describes the heart as an access point to a source of wisdom and intelligence that we can use to experience more balance, creativity, and intuitive capacities.

In the Western world, more credibility is given to the brain than the heart. Logical, rational thought is deemed more accurate and reliable than the wisdom contained in the heart. Did you know that the heart sends more information to the brain than the brain sends to the heart?

It also has the most powerful electromagnetic field in the body. It's about sixty times greater in amplitude than the electrical activity generated by the brain and can be detected nearly 1m away from the body. This means that people and pets in your immediate environment can be affected by the state of your heart. Maybe this explains why you feel so good in some people's company and not in others?

IT'S A MIRACLE TO ME THAT THIS OLD FUEL PUMP HAS BEEN TICKING OVER SINCE 1920. THANKS TO ITS UNFALTERING PERSEVERANCE, YET ANOTHER DAY HAS DAWNED THAT I'VE NEVER SEEN BEFORE.

SIR TOM MOORE

The heart is the gateway to compassion, gratitude, joy, peace, fulfilment, and happiness. Far from being soft, the heart has a strength that can guide us towards greater resilience, courage, and purpose. When we begin to see our hearts as a place to access inner guidance and wisdom, our worlds become more vibrant and interesting.

What does 'living from the heart' look like?

The relentless pace of modern life, our fear of uncomfortable emotions, and the stereotypes relating to what it means to be 'heart-centred', have resulted in an individual and collective disconnection from our hearts. When you begin to reconnect with this aspect of yourself, it's important to go gently. Imagine your heart is like a sleeping child. Pull back the covers and wake this wisdom centre softly. Trust that as you do, you will begin to feel more open and alive.

During my recovery, I began the process of waking my heart by simply pausing whenever I felt myself getting busy, overwhelmed, or caught inside my head. I'd take a few deep breaths and imagine them landing in my heart. If I was on my own, I'd place my hand on my chest and feel the warmth of my own skin. Amazingly, this simple physical gesture of placing my hand on my chest was enough to bring me down from my mind and relax my nervous system.

From here, I would open to any emotions that were arising. In truth, these emotions had probably been there a while, I was just too caught inside my head to notice them. I would offer these emotions (the overwhelm, fear, guilt, distraction, or worry) my attention. I would notice where they found a home in my body (often across my back or in my belly).

After just a few weeks of doing this short practice each day, I felt totally different. I was less stressed and more grounded and at ease. Excited about this new world that was emerging for me, I took the practice one step further. I began to ask my heart this simple question: *Heart, what message do you have for me, what would you have me know?*

My heart responded immediately (and had quite a sense of humour too!). Here are some of the things my heart has said to me over the years.

You are tired, have a rest.
Drink more water, your organs are thirsty.
Stop taking things so personally, not everything is about you.
Be kind to your body.
Stop eating meat.
Forgive, forgive, forgive.

When I began to live less from my mind and more from my heart, I achieved amazing things in all aspects of my life. I like to call it 'doing, but from a being state' or 'heart-centred productivity'. Learning to value your heart as a tool for guidance and wise action will help you live a more purposeful and balanced life. You can try the practice I just described, or the one that follows.

EXERCISE: WAKING YOUR HEART

Begin by finding somewhere comfortable to sit.

Place your focus on your breath and the steady flow of air as it enters and leaves your body.

Imagine that the air is travelling into your heart or chest.

Stay with this sensation of breath travelling in and out of your heart for about five breaths.

From this open state, you can invite compassion in.

Repeating silently in your mind:

May I be well. May I be happy.

You may like to offer this compassion to someone in your life.

Repeating silently in your mind:

May you be well. May you be happy.

We all have the capacity to connect more deeply with our hearts. When we do, the pathways of compassion, gratitude, perspective, and connection open within and around us. Being brave enough to move down from your mind into the wisdom of your heart is a fundamental practice when redefining happiness, one that we will come back to time and time again throughout this book.

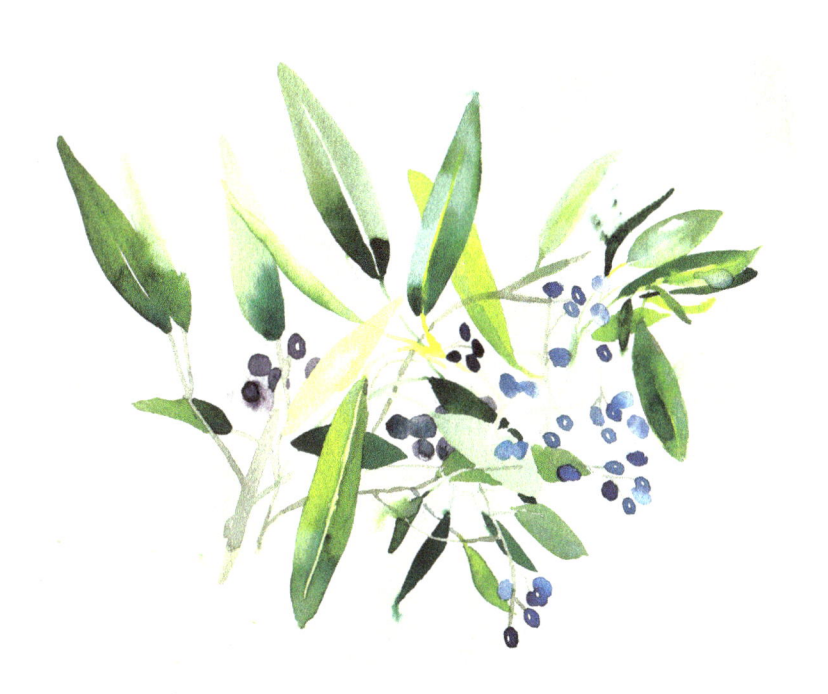

PATHWAY THREE: PERSPECTIVE

Learn to ask different questions

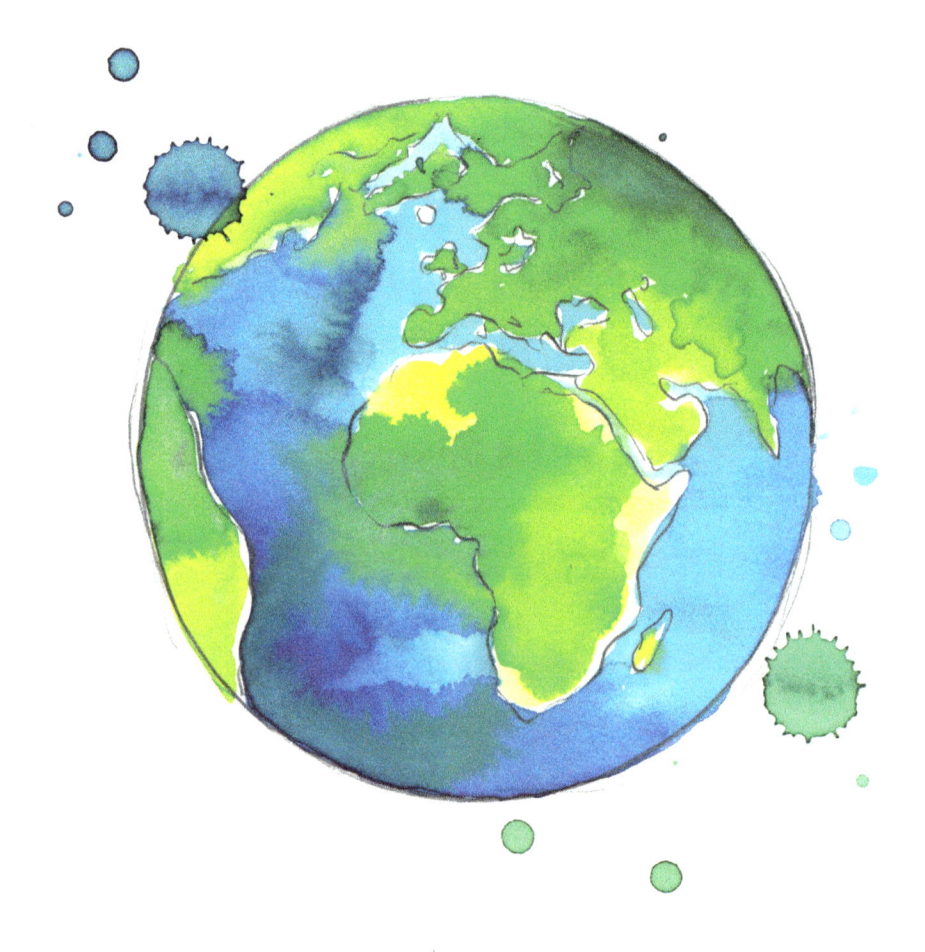

Ask questions that help you see things in new and liberating ways rather than confirm your own little stories and judgements.

It was Christmas Eve 1968 — the moment our collective relationship to planet Earth would change forever. On this night, the crew of the Apollo 8 spacecraft saw the Earth as no human had ever seen it before, rising above the barren moon in all its breathtaking beauty. The astronauts captured this image for all humans to see. In this now iconic photograph called *Earthrise*, planet Earth was the only thing in the entire universe that had any colour. Seeing our planet from this viewpoint altered our perspective and was a driving force of the environmental movement.

Astronauts from all different countries and professional backgrounds have expressed the powerful effect of seeing our planet from space. Collectively, they speak of a wave of awe and wonder that left them without words, a new appreciation for our fragile planet, the desire to protect and preserve, and to act for the good of all humanity.

This experience, of seeing Earth from space and being psychologically moved, is what Frank White, author and space philosopher, called the 'overview effect' (in his book of the same name). It is a powerful example of a mass collective perspective change. One of the biggest since Greek philosophers obtained empirical evidence that the world was a sphere and not flat.

Learning to broaden our perspective and to see things differently doesn't always need to feel like such a seismic shift in consciousness. It can look more like:

- A willingness to see other people's viewpoint.
- Noticing opportunities for growth and learning during hard times.
- Forgiveness of ourselves or others.
- An ability to shift from self-criticism to self-compassion.
- A desire to move from victim mode to empowered.

We all have the ability to see ourselves, our relationships, and our challenges in new and liberating ways. Neuroscience has confirmed that we can indeed 'teach an old dog new tricks', and that it's never too late to expand our thinking and change the way we show up in the world.

The great news is, if you're still here reading this book, then you've already begun to strengthen your neural pathways of perspective. Together, we've been letting go of old (and often limited) ways of seeing the world and replacing them with a set of beliefs that feel aligned to this more real and obtainable version of happiness.

Old thoughts / beliefs	*New thoughts / beliefs*
Happiness is a 'feel-good' state that includes the absence of pain, challenges, or uncomfortable emotions.	It's possible to be happy even amidst the setbacks and the challenges of adult life.
Pain should be avoided, pushed down, or hurried through.	We don't need to resist our pain. In fact, if we offer it our attention, it can provide us with greater confidence and purpose.
The challenges in my life are in some way my fault.	Everyone experiences hard times, it's just part of being human.
Self-compassion might make me unmotivated, lazy, or soft.	Self-compassion is an act of strength and will help me feel more resilient.
My mind always knows best.	The heart is intelligent. It can be helpful to check in with this part of me for guidance and direction.

Change the blame game

For years before my formal diagnosis, my pain felt all consuming and unpredictable. During this time, I was caught in a negative inner dialogue with my physical pain. When strong sensations would strike, I would immediately time travel into the past and ask myself: *What did I do to bring this on? Did I sit at the computer too long? Did I lift something too heavy?* The subtext to this line of questioning was that the pain episode was somehow my fault and that I had done something 'wrong' to cause it.

Sometimes, when the pain struck, my mind would travel to the future: *What if this pain lasts for ages? What if I'm in pain tomorrow when I've got that big meeting? What if it's still here on the weekend when I want to see my friends or play with my kids?* This line of questioning felt full of fear and apprehension.

The irony is that in the process of trying to understand my pain, I was making it worse for myself. World-recognised pain scientist Dr Beth Darnall confirms that this 'negative pain mindset' lights up the same regions in our brains that are involved in the processing of pain itself.

In my case, *and* for the 1.5 billion people who experience chronic pain every year, our negative thoughts are triggering the fear response, which in turn sets off our amygdala and amplifies our pain. The same can be said for other painful experiences. For example, when we add negative thoughts to our anxiety, job insecurity, or relationship status, we trigger the stress response and this makes the situation, and life, harder.

Realising that my thoughts were making my pain worse was a huge light-bulb moment for me. I immediately started to change my internal dialogue. At first, it felt hard to not go down the rabbit warren of 'trying to get to the bottom of my pain' (we humans love to have an answer). It also required great willpower to refrain from catastrophising about my future.

After a few months of managing my thoughts, I noticed a shift. I was moving from being desperate for a cure and a clear reason why I was in pain to a more spacious feeling of curiosity. It began to feel less like a relentless quest for 'the answer' and more like an invitation to surrender into the world of not knowing.

We think this 'not knowing' space is an abyss of darkness that will leave us feeling confused and afraid. But what I realised is that it feels like a relief to rest here for a little while. There is never one reason you are in physical, emotional, or mental pain (it's usually a collection of factors), and so taking a break from looking for something that doesn't exist feels good!

It's about your questions, not the answers

Learning to ask different questions was a key aspect of broadening my perspective and ultimately feeling less impacted by my pain. Moving from, *What did I do to bring this pain on?* to, *How can I support myself through this?* set the foundation for a new dynamic, one that recognised that nothing lasts forever and that there are gifts in unlikely places (we'll discuss impermanence more in the connection pathway).

Over time, my new line of questioning made me feel hopeful and less beholden to my pain. I felt less afraid. My pain was no longer an obstacle or something I thought was my fault. Instead, it became an opportunity to listen and respect my body, to connect with my inner determination, to receive support from family and friends, and to experience life more fully. Amazingly, when I let go of trying to control my pain, I felt more empowered.

I began to shift my perspective by reframing the questions I was asking myself.

For example:

Old Questions	*New Questions*
What did I do to bring the pain on?	What does my body need right now to feel better?
Why is this happening to me?	What is my body trying to tell me?
What if the pain this here tomorrow/next week/next year?	How can I bring myself back into the safety of the present moment?

Reframing is a tool that we can all use, whether we are dealing with chronic pain, a loss, disappointment, or any other daily challenge, big or small. I'm curious, when you receive 'negative feedback' at work, when your in-laws make a touchy comment, when a date or family gathering doesn't go to plan, what are the questions that swirl around in your mind?

Do these questions carry self-criticism, guilt, shame, or blame? Perhaps you can see how these questions are adding to your suffering (it's those second arrows again). Instead of searching for answers, try changing your line of questioning. It will bring you far more comfort and understanding.

Here are my three go-to questions I ask myself anytime I get all in my head about life:

1. What am I not seeing here (the perspective of others, an opportunity for growth, a hidden gift)?

2. How can I reframe this situation so that I feel less like a victim and more empowered?

3. What in this moment would offer me comfort?

The good news is you can change your perspective in an instant. Maybe you can remember a time you talked to a friend about a problem you were having and felt so much better afterwards, because of one comment they made. Perhaps you heard a piece of advice on a podcast that flipped your perspective. We can all do this for ourselves every day — if we start to ask the right questions.

EXERCISE:
OLD AND NEW QUESTIONS

Grab a pen and paper and try this writing exercise.

Begin by thinking about a challenge/situation you are facing that is causing you discomfort or stress. This may be a big life event like separation or job insecurity, or something small like a conversation that has left you feeling uncomfortable. Describe it in a few sentences.

Put two headings across the page: Old Questions and New Questions.

Write down at least three questions under each of the headings.

Notice how the new questions make you feel about yourself and the situation.

Let's talk toxic positivity

I know firsthand how annoying it can be when you are in the thick of a challenge and someone tells you to 'look on the bright side' or 'focus on the positive'. I can still remember the time an acquaintance asked me about the details of my pain. I explained that the pain was in my eyes, jaw, neck, shoulders, back, arms, hands, and hips. She responded chirpily, 'It's great that it's not in your legs and feet!'

Whilst this comment was true (sure, I was thrilled I could walk pain free, aren't you?), it wasn't helpful at that moment. Toxic positivity (the belief that no matter how dire or difficult a situation is, people should maintain a positive mindset) and gaslighting (when someone leads you to question your reality) are very different to the approach I'm suggesting — being brave enough to expand your perspective to see the hidden opportunities within your adversity.

The truth is, our challenges can result in significant loss and it's important to acknowledge these (and if possible, talk about them with people who don't want to brush them aside or paint them with positivity). For me, I had a list as long as my arm of the things I could no longer do or experience.

Perhaps, for you, it's the loss of financial security that comes from unstable work conditions and the dreams that die in the process. Maybe it's a loss of self-confidence or self-belief as a relationship ends and you find yourself alone. Or does the loss just come from getting older and knowing that there are certain life stages that will never be yours again?

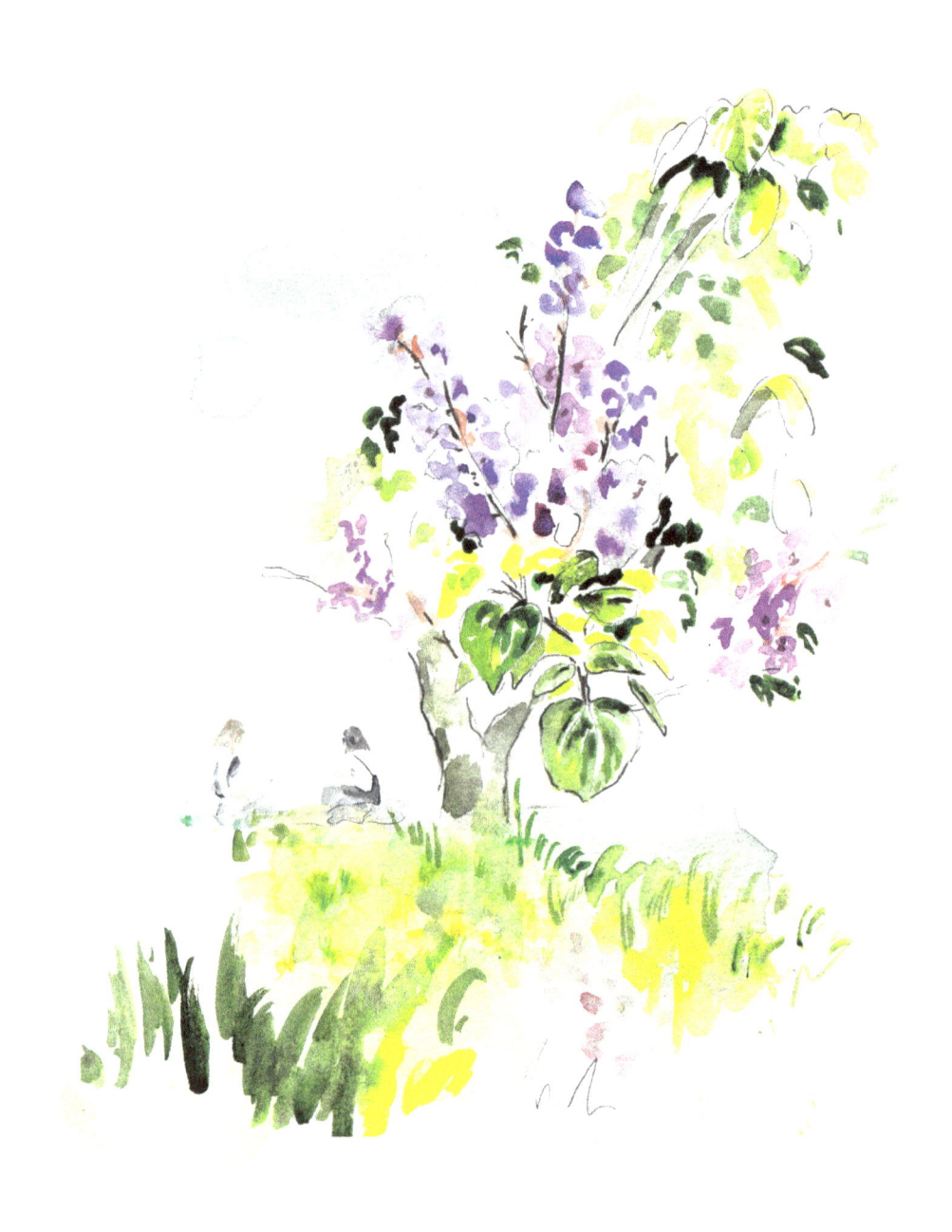

We need to offer ourselves a moment to really 'feel' these losses, to honour them before moving on. This doesn't require hours in therapy or a whole box of tissues — sometimes a few deep and compassionate breaths is enough. Next time you notice emotions around your loss coming up, pause and take a few deep breaths, place your hand on your heart, feel how soothing this can be. Perhaps say something to yourself like, *This feels really hard right now.*

Similarly, if you are talking to a friend who is going through a hard time, you can offer them this same moment of presence. You can breathe deep into your heart, really see them and what they are going through, and offer them similar words like, 'These are really big things you are navigating. I want you to know that I am here for you.' These simple words, this act of really 'seeing' your friend in their pain is worth more than any suggestion about how they could improve their lives.

Gift-wrapping our tough times

I know, I know, it sounds like a cliché: there's a gift in every challenge. But wouldn't you rather believe it than not? Plus, being willing to see the gifts within our challenges doesn't negate our losses. It simply acknowledges that we are complex human beings who can experience both grief and gratitude, loss and learning, at the same time.

In order to really experience the opportunities borne from adversity, we need to expand our definition of what constitutes a gift. We often think that the upside of our challenges needs to be happy and filled with relief, making you feel the way you do when you receive a present wrapped beautifully from a friend.

In truth, the gifts we receive from challenges often feel less high vibe and celebratory, and more subtle and grounding. After working with people all around the world to seek out the hidden jewels within their adversity, I've noticed that whilst the challenges can be unique, the gifts are often the same:

- Letting go of the need to be perfect.
- Letting go of the need to please everyone.
- Learning to prioritise rest, self-care, and compassion.
- Being able to ask for help from family and friends.
- Getting clear on what really matters.
- Learning to advocate for yourself and stand up for what you need and deserve.
- Facing your fears and realising that you are stronger than you ever imagined.

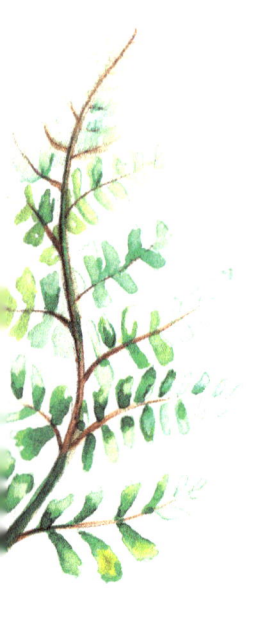

EXERCISE: THANKS FOR THE MEMORY!

With the passage of time, it becomes easier to see the gifts. So, it can be helpful to start by reflecting on a challenge that has long passed. Like the health scare that was a catalyst for you embracing a healthier and more stress-free lifestyle. Or the job you didn't get that encouraged you to study more or follow another avenue.

Find a comfortable place to sit and close your eyes.

Take a few deep breaths.

Allow a challenge from your past to surface. Really notice any memories, experiences, or sensations that emerge.

Be open to noticing that the pain you experienced in that moment is no longer present. That just like the clouds move across the sky, your challenges move in and out of your life also.

See if you can locate any hidden gifts or opportunities within this challenge. Perhaps in the form of heightened self-care, a change in life direction, or an increase in inner strength and resilience.

Offer this challenge a smile.

Acknowledge yourself for being willing to do this practice.

Trust that, as you strengthen your capacity to see the gifts in past challenges, it will become easier to see your present-moment adversities in this same way.

What's in a name?

I know I sounded like the fun police earlier when suggesting that the gifts we receive from our challenges aren't supposed to feel high vibe and celebratory. I'm all for having fun and not taking life too seriously. I also like to bring these feelings into my healing too.

About one year into my recovery, I decided to try a radical experiment. It was based on the quote by famous spiritual author Wayne Dyer: 'If you change the way you look at things, the things you look at change.' It consisted of me changing the name of my health diagnosis to see if it altered my experience.

Together, my kids and I brainstormed possible names for my condition. It reminded me of the two times we had come together to name our new puppies (minus the super cute balls of fluff at the end of the process). So, I said goodbye to fibromyalgia and hello to 'Teddy'. After just a few weeks, my experience changed. Here's what I noticed:

- Teddy isn't a doctor. He's not interested in the medical model of pain. So, when Teddy is around, I don't go down the path of thinking something is broken, torn, or out of place. I don't hurry off and make yet another doctor's appointment. Teddy reminds me not to outsource my healing, that I have the answers within.
- Teddy is soft, so every time he comes to visit, he reminds me to be soft (compassionate, gentle, and forgiving) with myself. This, in turn, reduces my stress and the cycle of pain.
- Teddy feels young and reminds me to get in touch with my inner child and my own capacity for healing.
- My three kids are more likely to ask me how Teddy is. This interest and open dialogue make me feel less alone.

- My kids feel less anxious when Teddy comes to visit. This means there is less tiptoeing around, less generalised anxiety, and a greater feeling of relaxation in my household.

This experiment got me thinking: *What else could be given a different name as a way of changing the experience?* Could we call our migraines Mary? Our backache Bob? Shall we refer to our inner critic as Indigo? Perhaps our worry wants to be called Wally the Warthog. *How could a simple name change alter our reactions?*

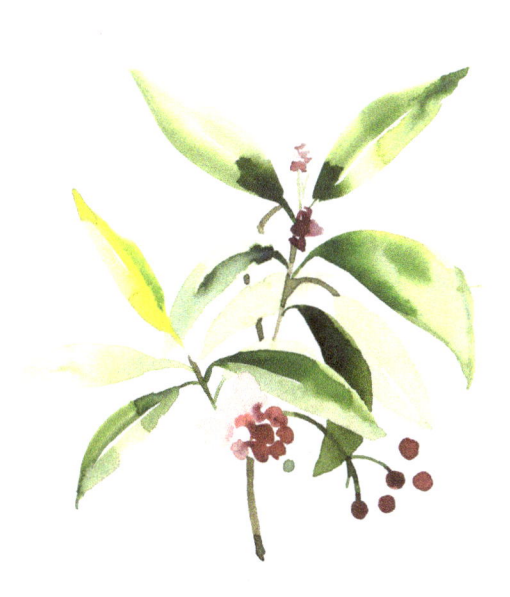

EXERCISE: RENAMING YOUR CHALLENGE

Grab a pen and paper. Think about a challenge, obstacle, or condition that you are currently facing.

Brainstorm as many new names as you can think of. The sillier the better! You can ask your family and friends for suggestions if you like. Notice how even this process is creating a feeling of lightness.

Pick one name from the list. Write down their characteristics, including personality, colour, shape, and feel (there are no right or wrong answers here).

Spend a few minutes imagining what might happen when you refer to your challenge in this way over a period of two weeks. Make a note of these possible side effects.

Keep this paper and refer to it in two weeks' time. Compare and contrast your experience. Make a note of all the ways your experience changed, hopefully for the better.

The wonders of your world

We've completed the full orbit and are back to where we began — at that image of our precious planet Earth, luminous amidst the backdrop of darkness. Making room for awe and wonder, allowing yourself the time and the space to be moved and humbled by the miracle that is each day on planet Earth is a crucial aspect of expanding your perspective and walking towards greater happiness.

When we reorientate our awareness towards the mystery (both in our challenges and our lives) and increase our tolerance for not having all the answers, we move away from the stories, judgements, and drama that keep us small, afraid, and unhappy.

In our Google-based world, where we have access to information twenty-four seven, we are experiencing what famous musician and songwriter Tom Waits refers to as 'a deficit of wonder'. When questions arise, we immediately turn to our screens in search of the answer. Doing this reduces our capacity to wonder, to meander within our minds, to imagine and create. So, what can we do instead? We can make awe and wonder a priority in our everyday lives.

The benefits of wonder are spelled out beautifully in the book *The Wonder Method, Energy Healing and The Art of Awakening Through Wonder* by Alain and Jody Herriotts and Tyler Odysseus. These include:

- Freeing yourself from the drama in your life.
- Experiencing more joy.

- Solving problems in unique ways.
- Using challenges as a vehicle for growth.
- Finding greater balance and happiness.

Philosophers, religious scholars, poets, and artists have been exploring awe and its capacity to change how we feel about ourselves and the world for centuries. Albert Einstein wrote in the book *Living Philosophies* that the most beautiful thing we can experience is the mysterious. He stated, 'He to whom this emotion is a stranger, who can no longer pause to wonder and stand rapt in awe, is as good as dead; his eyes are closed.'

More recently, psychologists and neuroscientists have shown an interest in the impact of awe and wonder on our everyday lives. A white paper prepared by The Greater Good Science Center at UC Berkeley entitled *The Science of Awe* provides a detailed overview of the research to date. The following six findings are particularly interesting and exciting:

1. Awe diminishes a person's sense of self, shifting their focus away from their own concerns.

2. Awe makes a person feel more humble. They can present a more balanced view of their strengths and weaknesses, and acknowledge the contribution of outside forces in their own personal accomplishments.

3. Awe encourages people to become less reliant on internalised scripts and more able to expand their thinking.

4. Awe encourages us to expand our perception of time, in so doing, we feel less pressured or starved for time.

5. Awe allows us to feel more connected to other people and humanity. It can encourage us to be more kind, compassionate, and giving.

6. Awe makes us less focused on the material aspects of our lives.

You don't need to travel to outer space in order to experience awe and wonder. Looking up at the night sky may be enough to elicit these feelings. Similarly, awe and wonder aren't only to be found in a forest full of one-hundred-year-old trees. You can find it by looking deeply into one leaf. It has more to do with the attention and intention you offer than the magnitude of the experience.

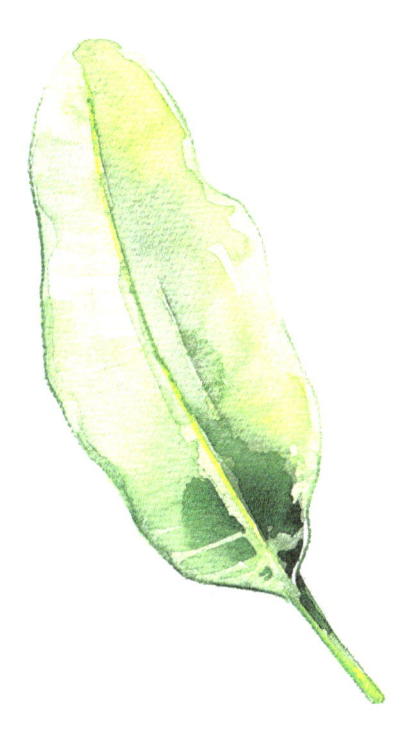

Seven ways to feel more awe-some

1. Notice the small details of the season you are in. Admire the perfect processes held in nature.

2. Sit somewhere green like a forest or park and immerse yourself in the sight and soundscape.

3. Take the time to witness a sunrise or sunset.

4. Look up at the stars and allow yourself to feel small but also part of the mystery.

5. Listen to music and admire the skill of the musicians. Allow the music to create emotion within you.

6. Visit an art gallery and allow your curiosity to run wild. Refrain from making judgements, and instead, allow yourself to be moved.

7. Spend time with a child. Notice their questions. Let their perspective rub off on you.

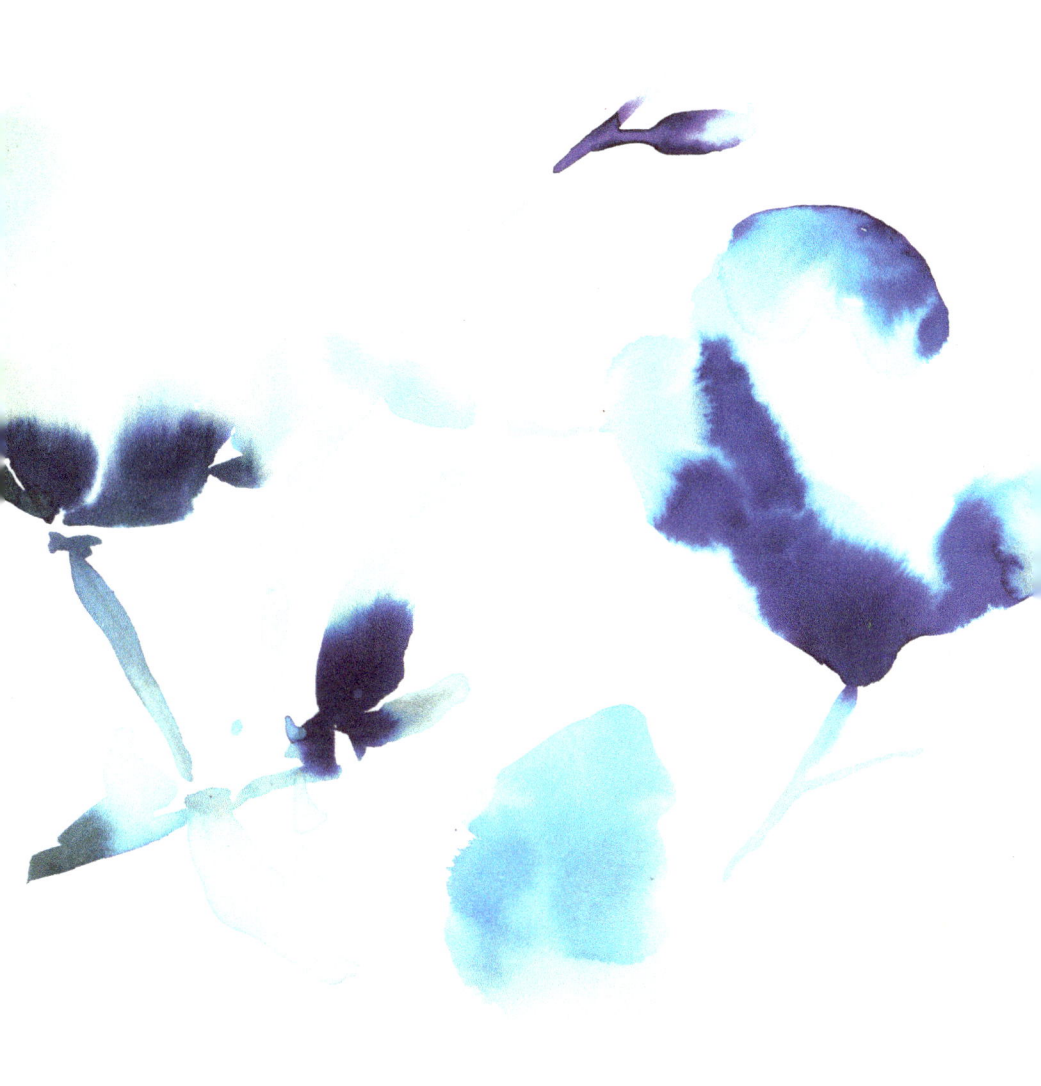

AWE IS A LIGHTNING BOLT THAT MARKS IN MEMORY THOSE MOMENTS WHEN THE DOORS OF PERCEPTION ARE CLEANSED AND WE SEE WITH STARTLING CLARITY WHAT IS TRULY IMPORTANT IN LIFE.

DAVID ELKINS

Redefining happiness includes changing the feel of the questions we ask ourselves daily. We must shift from trying to find a 'cure' for our metaphorical aches and pains to the more interesting landscape of curiosity. When we are brave enough to rest in the space of not knowing, we are more able to access the gifts within our challenges. Cultivating this curious beginner's mind also creates space for more fun, awe, and wonder. We begin to notice and be moved by everyday vistas that suddenly feel more vibrant and awe-some!

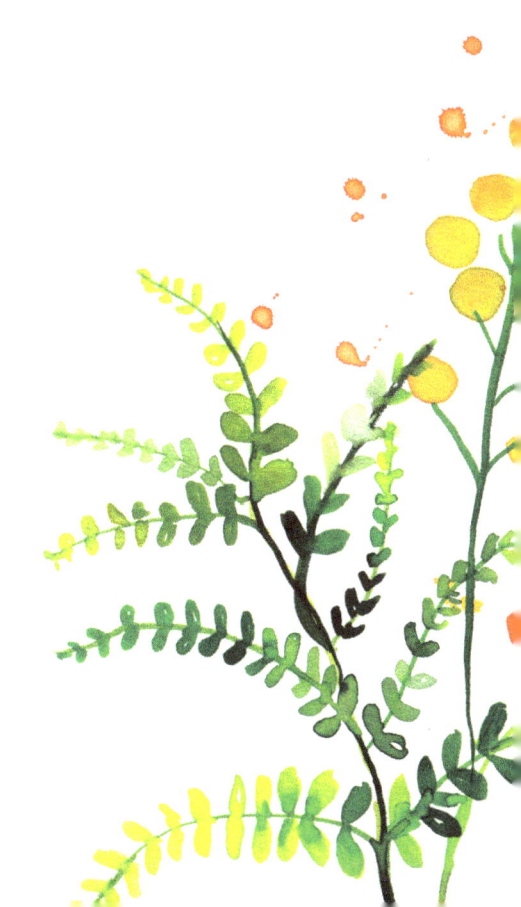

EXERCISE: BE MOVED BY THE MYSTERY

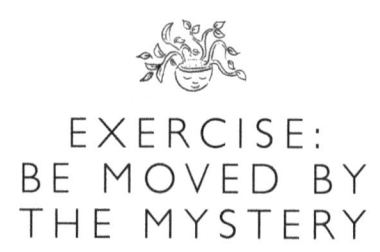

Art moves us beyond the rational thinking mind into the world of our heart. It can evoke a sense of awe and wonder within us.

Sit quietly and gaze at the illustration *Underwater Love* for one minute.

Breathe. Notice colours, shapes, and small details.

Allow emotions to swell.

Invite your perspective to expand.

Notice what opens up within you. Perhaps a desire to protect and preserve. A willingness to live life more fully. An urge to explore.

Take one deep breath into this moment of possibility.

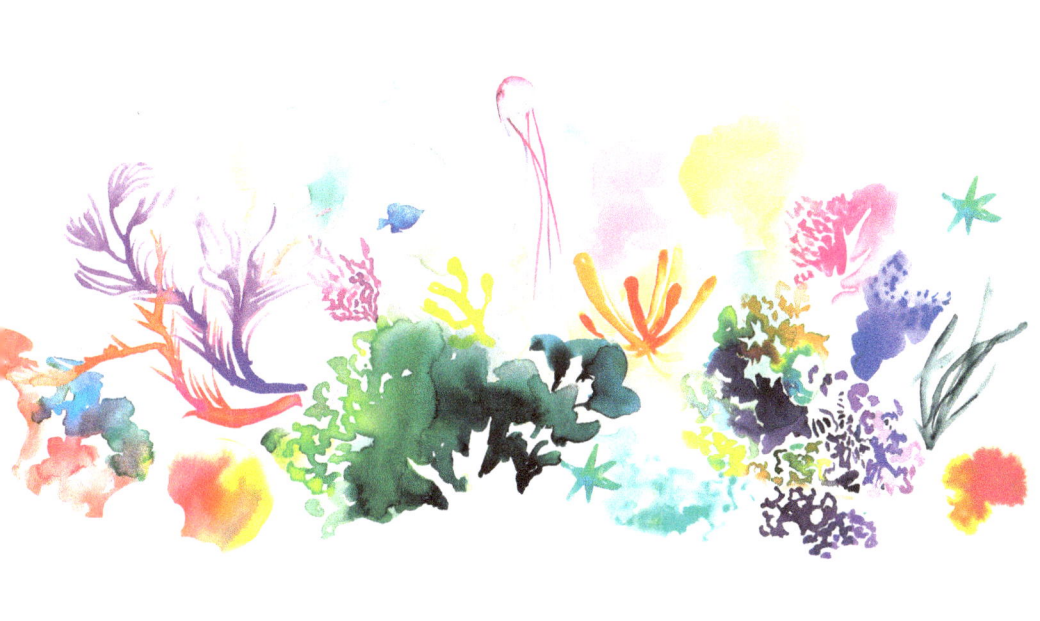

PATHWAY FOUR: GRATITUDE

The simpler, the better

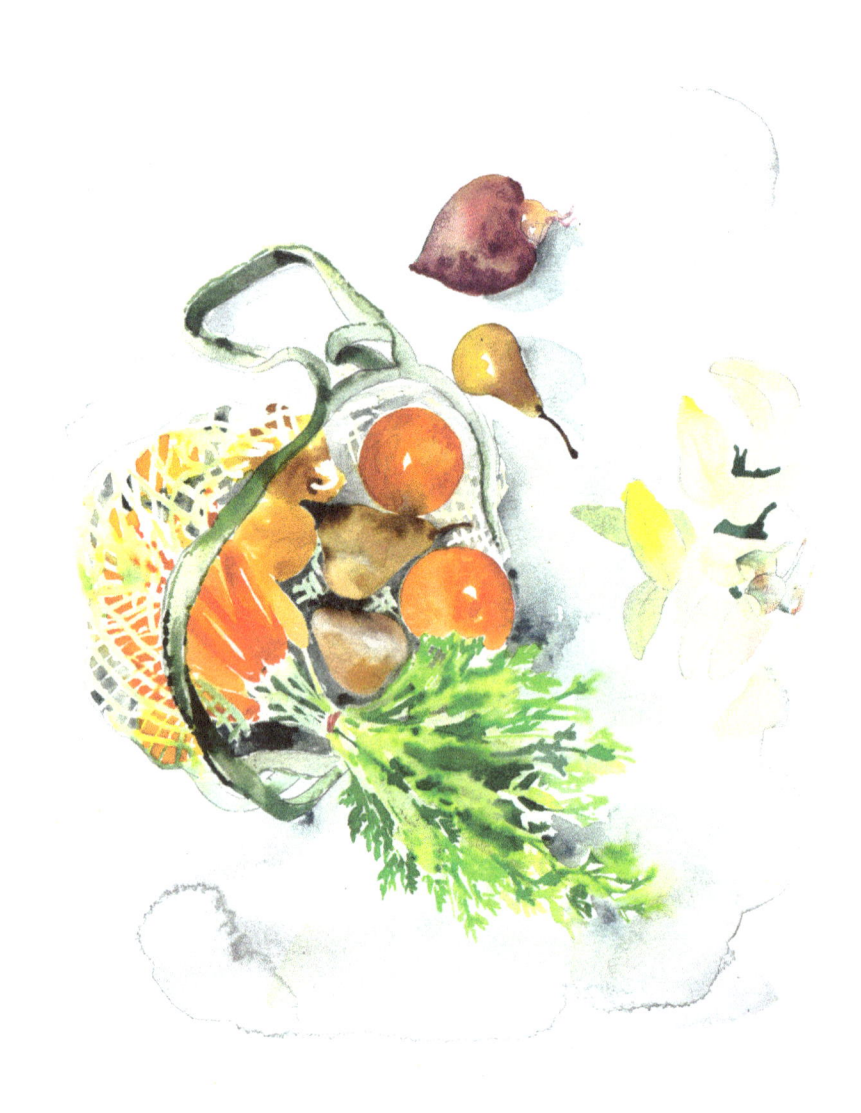

For gratitude to contribute to your wellbeing and happiness, you need to linger in these moments long enough for them to actually land.

Ah, gratitude, what can I say that hasn't already been printed as a quote in a diary or shared on social media (#grateful)? The sad truth is that this pathway for happiness has been so overdone in popular culture that we are numb from overexposure. For many of us, we're tired of gratitude before we've really given it a go or experienced it at a deeper level.

Much like compassion, gratitude's power lives not as words on paper, but as an energy that begins in the heart and then radiates out into our bodies, lives, and relationships. Gratitude 'works' best when it arises naturally from the wellspring within, not from our own guilt *(I should be more grateful)* or from the urgings of family, friends, or well-meaning strangers on social media ('Practice gratitude, it will change your life!').

Gratitude is for everyone, not just people who have a naturally optimistic or positive disposition. We can all learn to be moved by the simple joys in life, no matter our age, life stage, or circumstance. It's possible for each of us to pause and savour a small, precious moment: a delicious meal, laughter with a friend, a hug that lasted longer than you expected, your dog's excitement as you return from work, or a ray of sunshine on a cloudy morning.

So, perhaps instead of asking ourselves, *How do I become more grateful?* We could get curious and enquire, *What gets in the way of me and my naturally grateful self?*

Ask yourself these simple questions as a way of exploring this idea:

- Are you just too busy? (Subtext — you prioritise getting things done over pausing to appreciate the small things — sorry but ouch!)
- Do you tell yourself you'll make time for gratitude when everything else is done (that final email sent, dishes cleaned, and the washing put away)?
- Are you desensitised to gratitude, having scrolled past one too many quotes on social media?
- Do you think gratitude is for overly positive, optimistic, or happy people (and that's not you)?
- Do you feel like gratitude is only for special occasions — like holidays, dinners out, or birthdays, not for the ordinary everyday moments of life?
- Do the high expectations you place on yourself and others take your focus away from appreciation?

When we prioritise achievement over experience or productivity over pleasure, low-level stress builds and as a result, our in-built negativity bias (our tendency to pay more attention to perceived threats rather than opportunities) becomes more pronounced.

Our focus becomes fixated on just getting through the day; meetings, emails, heavy traffic, shopping lists, and dirty dishes become our world. From this vantage point, we just can't see (or feel moved by) the ordinary wonders and delight of everyday life. Making a commitment to be more grateful sets in motion a process for changing the way we experience life. We move from expectation to appreciation.

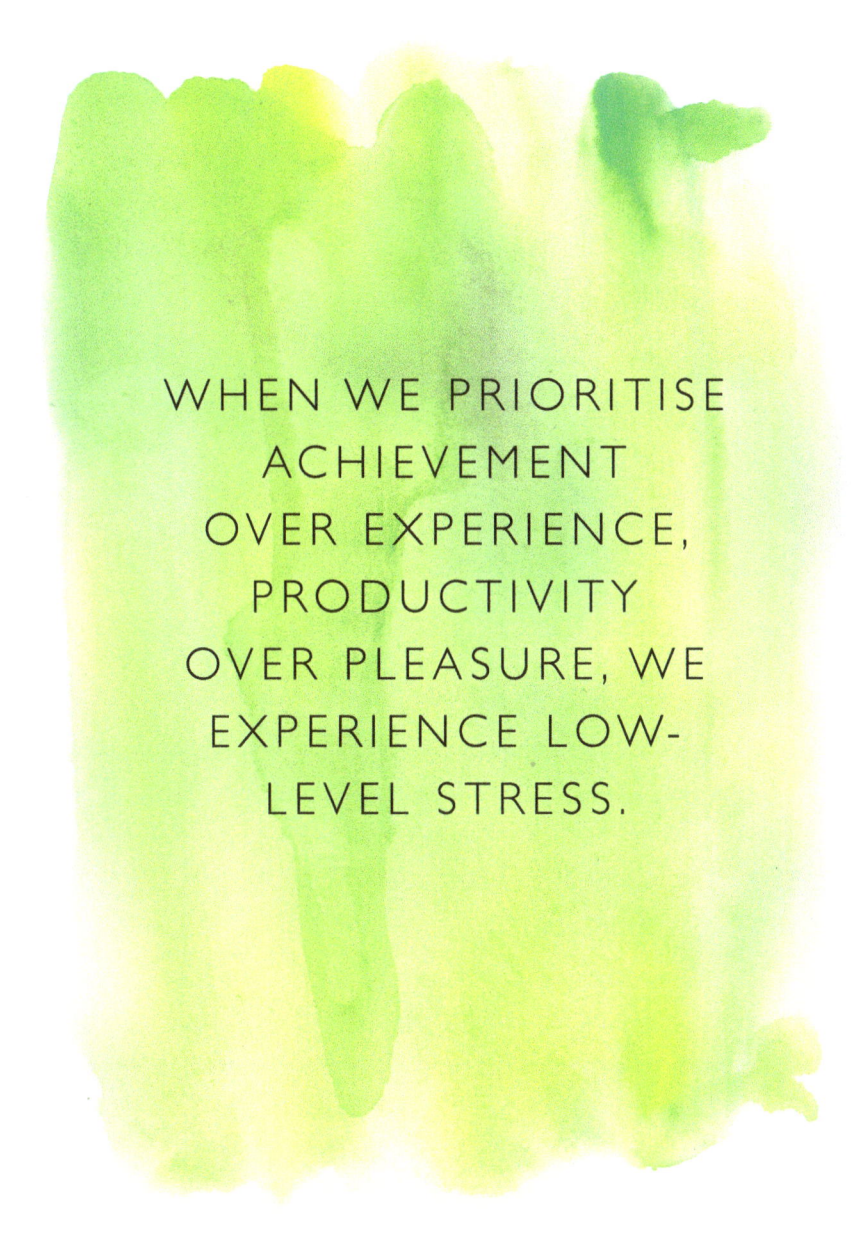

WHEN WE PRIORITISE ACHIEVEMENT OVER EXPERIENCE, PRODUCTIVITY OVER PLEASURE, WE EXPERIENCE LOW-LEVEL STRESS.

Here are my top three practices to increase my appreciation.

Appreciation for connection

After catching up with a friend, before I check my phone and move onto the next thing, I take one minute to have a grateful moment. I reflect on how good it felt to connect, to laugh, to feel seen and heard. I notice any softening in my body or warmth in my heart. I trust that this small moment will help the experience of friendship and connection land on my nervous system.

Appreciation for my children

When I'm with my kids, perhaps walking the dog or just chatting whilst in the car, I tell them how much I enjoy their company and how happy I feel in the moment. Depending on their age, I might share how it feels in my heart or what I like about their personality. Being verbal about the grateful moment has the double benefit of deepening my experience and modelling gratitude and connection to my children.

Appreciation for this moment

When I have my morning coffee, I purposefully don't look at my phone. Instead, I engage all my senses. I play a game with myself to stay present until all the heat has left the mug (you'd be surprised how long it stays warm!).

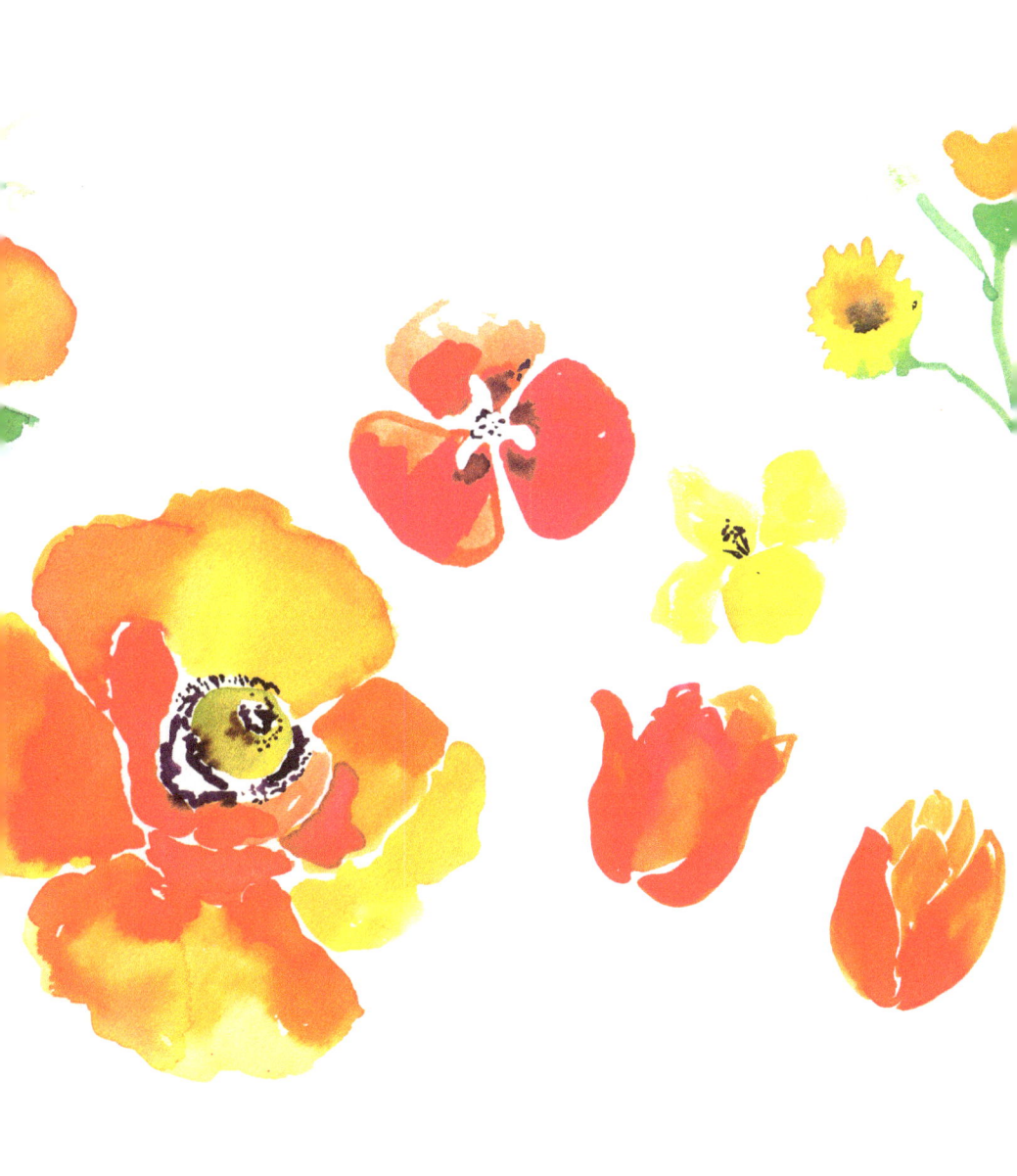

Gratitude 101 — what they didn't teach you at school

Unfortunately, many of us weren't taught at school *how* to practice gratitude (the good news is that this is changing in schools today). So, for many of us, even when we do try to be more grateful, the experience falls short. It doesn't feel as good as we imagined, and we are left wondering what all the gratitude hype is about.

Perhaps these scenarios sound familiar:

- You make an effort to enjoy the first sip of your morning smoothie, juice, tea, or coffee, noticing how good it tastes but then drink the remainder whilst scrolling through your emails or social media.
- A beautiful tree or flower in bloom catches your eye, but instead of taking a moment to really notice the colours, details and how they make you feel, you go back to the mental trance that is planning for tomorrow.
- As you take your evening shower, you feel the warm water on your skin for a moment, but before long, your focus turns to replaying your day and all the things you didn't get done.

For a grateful moment to have a lasting impact on our emotional wellbeing, we need to 'let the moment land'. Chances are, unless someone tells you this important piece of information, you are probably moving on from the moment too quickly.

If you only take one thing from this book, let it be the importance of lingering, of letting moments (of gratitude, calm, compassion, connection, vitality …) land. This is when experiences turn from what neuroscientists call 'a fleeting state' to 'a lasting trait'. In other words, we move from experiencing a grateful moment to being a grateful person.

The best part is, when these qualities become in-built and part of who we are, it's easier to have even more of these moments, and so the positive cycle continues.

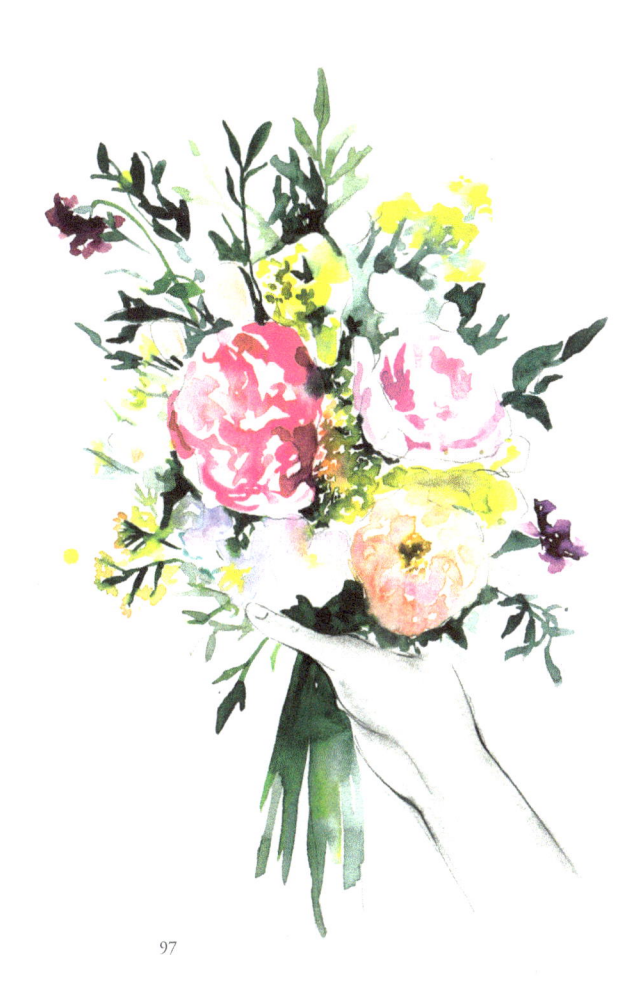

EXERCISE: LETTING GRATITUDE LAND

You can do this in the moment, when you are experiencing something pleasant, or later whenever you need a gratitude boost. Given that our brains don't distinguish between past, present, and future visualisations, it's possible to practice letting gratitude land by recollecting a moment from your past or imagining a moment in your future.

Begin by finding somewhere comfortable to sit.

Close your eyes and take three deep breaths.

Open to a feeling of gratitude for the simple act of breathing. Each inhale is an opportunity to invite in fresh oxygen. Each exhale is an opportunity to rid your body of carbon dioxide.

Ask yourself one of these three questions:

1. What past moment am I grateful for?
2. What am I grateful for in my life right now?
3. What future possibility am I grateful for?

Trust whatever emerges.

Stay with this memory/situation/possibility of gratitude for five deep breaths.

You may like to imagine that you are breathing the feeling of gratitude into your body. You can focus on physical sensations or emotions, or any feelings in your heart. Offer whatever emerges a smile.

Well done, you just let a moment of gratitude land.

You don't need to be sitting still with your eyes closed in order to really let moments land, you can explore this practice anywhere, anytime.

From expectation to appreciation

Gratitude isn't about pretending the tough times aren't tough, layering your pain with false positivity or putting on a brave face. It's more about acknowledging that, even in the hard times, we always have something to be grateful for, in at least one area of our lives: work, relationships, family, health, or finances.

If you are finding your toddler, teenager, or partner particularly challenging, don't put pressure on yourself to focus your gratitude in their direction. Instead, you could allow it to land on another aspect of your life: your friendships, your pet, your full fridge, or the flowers and plants in your garden.

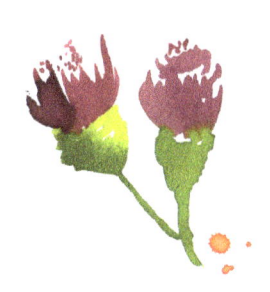

Gratitude elicits the most warmth (and makes us happier) when it's directed at our relationships, experiences, or the simple things that we often take for granted. In other words, focus your gratitude on people more than possessions: simple moments rather than big milestones.

In our busy lives, it's often the simple things that we take for granted. Like how our body breathes all day, every day, keeping us alive. Our head hits the pillow at the end of the day, and of course, we just expect that our body will continue to breathe as we sleep. This energy of expectation shields us from a sense of appreciation for the miracle that is each breath.

During the global pandemic, when COVID-19 put pressure on our lungs and we were required to wear masks and spend large periods of time inside, the preciousness of our lungs and fresh air became crystal clear. What we had once taken for granted transformed into something we cherished and wanted to protect.

EXERCISE: THE SIMPLE THINGS

Find somewhere comfortable to sit or stand and take three grateful breaths. Take a moment to consider:

You will breathe approximately 22,000 times today and 8 million times this year.

Your lungs contain approximately 2,400km of airways.

Breathing is the most important thing your body does.

When you breathe in oxygen it helps defend your immune system, increases cognitive clarity, and regenerate cells.

You can use your breath to alter your heart rate and your nervous system.

The fastest way to relax your body, reduce anxiety or overwhelm is to extend your exhale.

The fastest way to feel more energised is to extend your inhale.

When you focus on your breathing, you are immediately transported into the present moment.

Enjoy three more grateful breaths.

Now see how you feel!

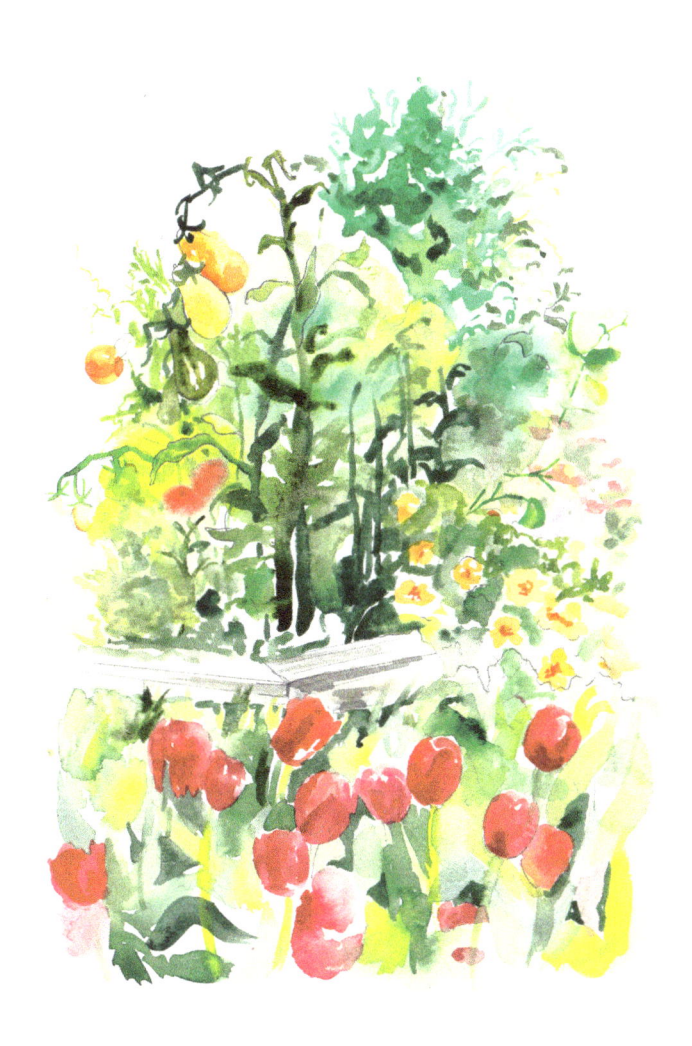

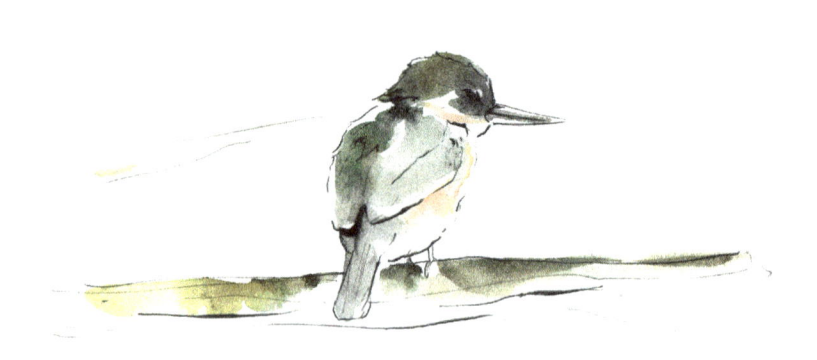

Thank you breath,
for carrying the sweet song of birds into my mornings,
for the rustle you make when weaving through the tall trees.
Thank you for moving the wispy white clouds across our clear blue sky,
for the delight you bring as you cool my skin on a hot summer's day,
for drying my clothes on the line.
Thank you for encouraging the autumn leaves to dance as they fall,
for carrying the hopeful seeds in spring,
for the winter's howl that whispers it's time to look within.
Thank you for sustaining me,
for connecting me to all life,
to the blue whales in Antarctica, the leopards in the Serengeti, and the earthworms in my garden.

Dear breath, see my body as your next adventure,
fill my lungs with fresh oxygen, nutrients, and life force,
find refuge for a moment in my heart.
And breath, if your curiosity is sparked,
may you explore the hidden pockets of me,
the parts I so often judge or ignore.
May you soothe these parts of me from the ache of being forgotten, of not being enough.
Precious breath, paint my entire body with beginnings,
so that I may feel inspired and alive.

Aging gratefully

We live in a world where being young is beautiful and aging is something to fear or resist. We receive both strong and subtle messages from social media, advertising, friends, and family about how our bodies should look and what they should be able to do. These external pressures often lead to us having an unhealthy relationship with our bodies. We get caught in the habit of wishing our bodies looked different or could still do the things they used to, like run long distances, stay up late, or eat hot chips or cake without gaining weight.

How we felt about ourselves during childhood and adolescence may also contribute to this dynamic. If we felt uncomfortable in our bodies growing up, or if we received messages from family or friends that we were too chubby or too skinny, we can take these insecurities into our adult lives. We end up yo-yo dieting, following the latest fitness fad, or changing our hair in the subconscious hope that we'll be loved and accepted if we look a certain way.

When we interact with our bodies in these more limited and self-critical ways, we are missing the bigger picture: that our bodies are miraculous!

Limited Perspective	*Grateful Perspective*
My skin looks old, blemished, wrinkled or untoned.	My skin is an incredible organ that protects me from toxins, radiation and harmful pollutants. It's not old because every twenty-eight days it renews itself completely.
I'm not as strong, fit or flexible as I used to be.	Within my body there are over six hundred different muscles that help me live a full life. My body is strong. Gram for gram, my bones are stronger than steel.
My body feels heavy and tired. It's full of aches and pains.	My body is dynamic, every second it's producing 25 million new cells. It's constantly rejuvenating and healing.
I'm so tired of dealing with my obsessive thoughts: the worries, ruminations and regrets.	My brain is amazing, it's always taking in raw information and giving it meaning so my life makes more sense. I can retrain my brain to focus on more positive aspects of my life.

Over the seven years I was caught in the debilitating cycle of chronic pain, I went from being fit and active, running, playing tennis, swimming, and lifting weights, to not even being able to grate a carrot, hold a bag of groceries, or drive the car.

I know firsthand what it feels like to be frustrated and let down by your body. In these dark times it takes courage to reorientate your awareness away from disappointment towards gratitude. We must remember, it's during these times we need gratitude the most.

It's important, however, to distinguish between *feeling* grateful and *being* grateful. When times are tough you don't need to 'manufacture' a feeling of gratitude. Instead, you can shift your awareness to being grateful. In my case, for all the miraculous things my body was still able to do — like walk, breathe, regenerate, sense, and feel.

Whatever concern, disappointment, or insecurity you have about your body, you can benefit from this simple practice of shifting your awareness away from your body's perceived flaws and limitations towards a sense of appreciation and thankfulness.

EXERCISE: GRATEFUL BODY SCAN

Find yourself a quiet place to sit. Take a few deep breaths.

Read the lines below out loud or in your mind.

Take a deep breath between each line and really let the words land in your body, mind and heart.

Thank you mind, for helping me make sense of the world, for allowing me to learn new things, broaden my perspective, and solve problems creatively.

Thank you eyes, for allowing me to see the faces of those I love, the colour of the sky at sunset, and the familiar features of my neighbourhood.

Thank you ears, for offering me the gift of music, laughter, and the words spoken by family, friends, and the people I admire.

Thank you mouth, for allowing me to taste and enjoy all different types of food.

Thank you chest, for knowing exactly how to receive each breath, for taking in fresh oxygen and ridding my body of carbon dioxide.

Thank you heart, for beating, feeling, loving, and reminding me what is true in this world.

Thank you legs, for taking me where I want to go, for allowing me to move forward in the direction of what truly matters and away from things that aren't important.

Thank you hands, for helping me carry, hold, embrace, and express myself.

Thank you body, for working all day, every day like a complex but beautiful orchestra, so that I can experience the miracle that is each day on planet Earth.

In his book, *Gratitude,* bestselling author and professor of neurology Oliver Sacks shares his reflections on completing a life and coming to terms with his own death. He explains:

> *'My predominant feeling is one of gratitude. I have loved and been loved; I have been given much and have given something in return; I have read and travelled and thought and written ... Above all, I have been a sentient being, a thinking animal, on this beautiful planet, and that in itself has been an enormous privilege and adventure.'*

Like Oliver Sacks, may you also have the courage to weave gratitude through your days.

Remembering the hard times

When we commit to making gratitude a daily practice, it becomes easier to experience gratitude for the myriad of human experiences, even the ones that feel hard.

Take a moment to consider how those hard times you made it through help you to feel more grateful for your life right now.

- Perhaps that difficult break-up and period of loneliness has made you more appreciative of your current relationship and the moments of love and connection.
- Maybe that health crisis allowed you to really value the good health you are now experiencing.
- Did those times when your children were young make you grateful for the freedom you now experience as your kids are older and more independent?

- Maybe that period when work was stressful and unrewarding has allowed you to feel more grateful for your current job and the way it satisfies you?

In his book, *Thanks!*, Robert Emmons (one of the world's leading gratitude experts) explains how this contrast between 'how difficult life used to be' and 'how far we have come' elicits gratitude. Our minds like to make comparisons, and when we can contrast the present with negative times from our past, a feeling of gratitude and happiness builds within us.

In the previous chapter on perspective, we explored receiving the gifts from our challenges. Learning to be grateful for what arises out of hard times is another aspect of walking alongside our pain and growing through our adversities.

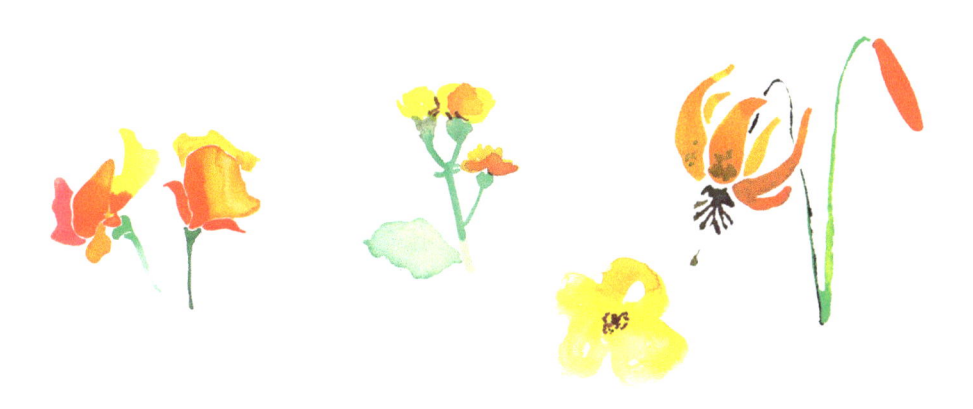

EXERCISE: HOW FAR YOU'VE COME

Grab a pen and paper. Take a moment to think back to a hard time in your life.

Describe it in a few sentences. Respond to each of these questions:

1. What lesson did this experience teach me?
2. What skills/capacities did I grow through this?
3. How does this moment make me feel more appreciative of my current life?

Take a moment to acknowledge how far you've come!

Gratitude in action

When I think back to the moments in my life when I've experienced deep gratitude, one Christmas comes to mind and heart. My three children were young (four, five, and seven years old). Family life was busy but full of love. There were Christmas presents to buy, kid's concerts to attend, an endless stream of social gatherings, and work to finish off. Amidst it all, I took the time to write two gratitude letters (if I'm totally honest, they were emails).

The first letter was to my meditation teacher. I shared how gaining my meditation qualification had given me a new sense of purpose and direction. I expressed my gratitude for the way he had so freely shared his knowledge and wisdom and for the gift that was his down-to-earth and often humorous teaching style.

The second letter was to my children's sports coach. I shared how appreciative I was for having him as a positive role model in my children's lives and the delight that I experienced seeing my kids grow in confidence.

Six years later, I look back at that Christmas period and cannot remember who I talked to at those social gatherings or whether I tidied up all my work commitments before the year was out. Nor can I remember what presents my kids received or whether the turkey was delicious or dry!

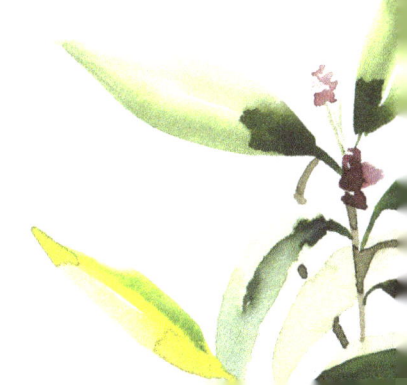

What I can remember (as clearly as if it were yesterday), are the two emails I received in return. I can recall the wave of positive emotion that washed over me as I read the two teachers' emails. This moment of connection, this willingness to acknowledge that our lives are made better by other people, was both humbling and energising. It made me feel alive.

In their letters, both teachers shared with me a sad truth; that these notes of appreciation arrive less frequently than you would imagine. I remember thinking how strange this was (as I knew how many other meditation students and parents were grateful for these two people). So, we find ourselves back where we began, asking ourselves once more: *What gets in the way of me and my naturally grateful self?*

It's so easy to not share our gratitude for others. Sure, we can blame it on being busy. We can tell ourselves there wasn't enough time to write a letter. I would argue however, that something deeper is at play. You see, writing a letter of gratitude involves a certain level of vulnerability as it includes really acknowledging the impact another has had on your life.

In our individualised culture where we are taught to be self-sufficient and independent, this level of intimacy and connection can feel uncomfortable. Taking off our mask of independence can feel scary, but when we do, we are rewarded with great moments of connection, gratitude, and ultimately, belonging.

EXERCISE: WRITE A GRATITUDE LETTER (AND REALLY MEAN IT!)

Before you sit down to express your thanks, take a few deep breaths into your heart. (We practised waking our hearts in the compassion chapter, remember?)

Remind yourself that writing this letter isn't another item on your to-do list, or something that you *should do* out of obligation. As Seneca, the Roman philosopher, explains in his book, *Letters from a Stoic,* 'We weigh not the bulk of the gift, but the quality of the goodwill which prompted it.'

Choose someone you feel grateful for, they may be someone in your life right now or someone from your past. In your own unique way, express your gratitude and appreciation.

Offer yourself a smile for moving beyond the 'I'm too busy' excuses towards a deeper experience of gratitude and connection.

Bonus points if you send the letter or email it to them!

PATHWAY FIVE: CALM

Don't tell me to relax

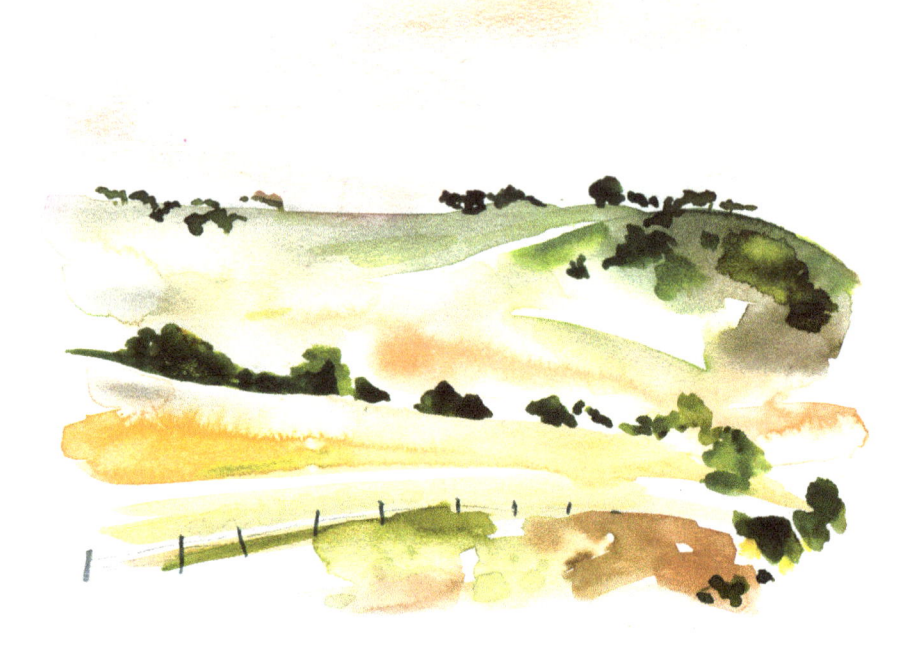

Learn to fall in love with all the different ways you can soothe your nervous system.

As we discussed in the gratitude pathway, the human body is complex and supremely intelligent. It is constantly responding to external stimuli and adjusting in order to keep us safe. One way it does this is through our autonomic nervous system. This system has two branches that are the mirror opposite of one another.

The 'sympathetic branch' upregulates our physiology, increasing our heart rate and our breathing, and pumping adrenaline and cortisol into our bloodstream. This is often referred to as fight, flight, or freeze, the stress response, the doing state, or the red zone.

Historically, this state was only triggered when there was a threat to our physical safety (perhaps a lion prowling in the distance). In our modern lives the stress response can get activated when we are rushing from task to task, trying to please everyone, or striving to meet our self-imposed high standards.

In contrast, the 'parasympathetic branch' of our autonomic nervous system downregulates our physiology, slowing our heart rate, our breathing, and returning our systems back to normal functioning. You may have heard this state being referred to as rest and digest, the relaxation response, the being state, or the green zone.

We can move into this state intentionally by taking a few deep breaths, lengthening our exhale, engaging our senses, and focusing on the present moment.

What colour is happiness?

Whilst both states are necessary for our survival, many of us spend too much time doing (red zone) and not enough time being (green zone). Given that real and sustainable happiness is found in the being state, it's no surprise that over time, prolonged periods in the red zone lead to physical, emotional, and psychological distress.

So how do you regain more balance between these two states so that you can feel happier from the inside out?

As we learnt in chapter one, the first step in change is awareness. So, let's begin by becoming aware of the key characteristics of the red and the green zones. From here, you'll be able to identify what zone you are in at different times throughout your day.

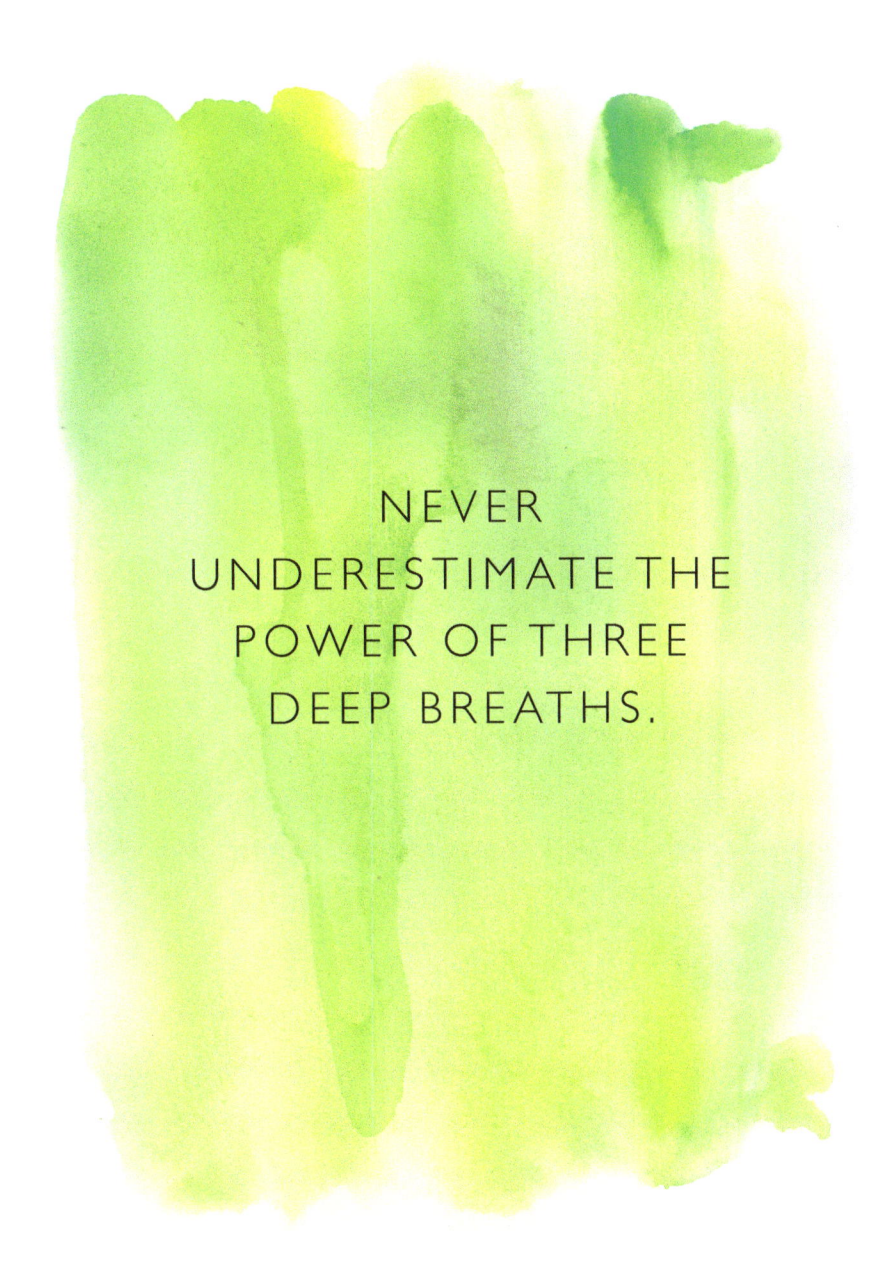

NEVER UNDERESTIMATE THE POWER OF THREE DEEP BREATHS.

Doing State / Red Zone

Thoughts are mainly focused on the past or the future.

You might feel scattered, like your thoughts are all over the place, or that you are 'in your head'.

You are focused on getting through your to-do list.

Your perspective narrows. You have specific ideas about the way things should be. This might feel like 'holding on', or judging yourself or others when things don't go to plan.

You think a lot about the small details of your life.

You get caught in the habits of striving, craving, or wanting more (this may relate to food, alcohol, exercise, social media, money, success, or even fun).

Your body may feel tense, tight, or sore. You may experience physical pain, recurring injuries, or migraines.

You often plan, strategise, or rehearse your future.
OR
You ruminate about the past, wishing things had turned out differently or that you had acted in another way.

Your emotions feel strong. They may take you by surprise or feel too big to handle. You may ignore or resist them.

Being State / Green Zone

Thoughts are focused on the present.

You might feel more settled and less 'in your head'.

You are focused on moments, experiences, and your relationships.

Your perspective broadens. You are more flexible in how things *should* be. This might feel like 'letting go'. You are more able to welcome the opinions of other people.

You are happy to 'go with the flow' and not worry about the little things.

You feel satisfied and content.

Your body feels relaxed, open, and at ease.

You can be present for the people, places and emotions that are right here, right now.

Your emotions feel manageable. You feel able to identify and acknowledge them.

What did you notice as you read through that list? Are you surprised how much time you spend in the red zone?

Take a moment to consider these questions:

- Does life feel easier when you are able to see the bigger picture, take things less personally, and acknowledge the opinions of others?
- Does time with your family or friends feel more enjoyable when you put down your phone, switch off from work, and just 'be in the moment'?
- Does your long to-do list sometimes make you feel stressed or scattered? From here, do things often fall through the cracks?
- Do you feel happier when you can identify your striving or perfectionist habits, take a deep breath, let go, and focus on the present moment?
- Do you feel more balanced and at ease when you notice your emotions before they get strong and feel out of control?

Cultivating happiness by finding a healthy balance between the red and the green zones will look and feel different for each of us. Some people can 'handle' longer periods in the red zone before they begin to experience stress and need to intentionally shift into the green zone. Others will have less tolerance for the red zone and will feel overwhelmed after only short periods of time in this state.

You may also have different tolerances for the red zone at different times in your life. I've heard mothers from all around the world say that before children they could tolerate stress, but now — with little sleep or alone time to recalibrate — these challenging moments hit them harder.

During the years of pandemic living, you may have noticed your capacity for the red zone diminished. Maybe you can think back to a time when a small event tipped you into a stressed state — a news story, a government response, or yet another change in COVID-19 guidelines. If you can identify with these situations, don't be hard on yourself — see them as a gift from your intelligent body, nudging you back into a being way of living.

Our capacity for the red zone has little to do with our resilience and inner strength and more to do with our unique nervous systems and personal histories. So if you have a nervous system that is sensitive or highly responsive to external stimuli, it's likely that you will really 'feel' too much time in the red zone.

You might experience physical pain or strong and uncalibrated emotions like fear, guilt, shame, or remorse. Maybe anxiety or insecurity creeps in. Perhaps a desire to hide away from the world or procrastinate presents itself after too much time in the red. If you have a history of trauma, burnout, or illness, or if you identify as an empath or 'highly sensitive person', your tolerance for the red zone may also be lower and that's okay too.

An important aspect of my recovery from chronic pain was befriending my sensitive nervous system. I became an 'expert' at noticing when I had moved into the red zone (using the descriptions in the previous table). Being able to identify the thoughts, emotions, and physical sensations I was experiencing in the context of my nervous system helped me take a step back and be more objective.

With this awareness came space and ultimately freedom to reframe the inner narrative about my illness. I let go of the story that I experienced chronic pain because I got stressed easily, wasn't resilient, or coping well enough with the daily challenges of life. Instead, I welcomed a new narrative which acknowledged that my pain stemmed from my unique physiology. No judgement. No blame. Expanding my perspective also reduced the second arrows of suffering that we explored in the compassion pathway — that the pain was somehow my fault.

It's empowering to learn how to use your nervous system to respond more skilfully to life's challenges and setbacks. Befriending your nervous system allows you to have more perspective and to feel less pulled in by the drama. It also softens those harmful second arrows. Remember, all you need to do is pause and take three deep breaths (long exhale), and you'll be ready to respond from the green zone.

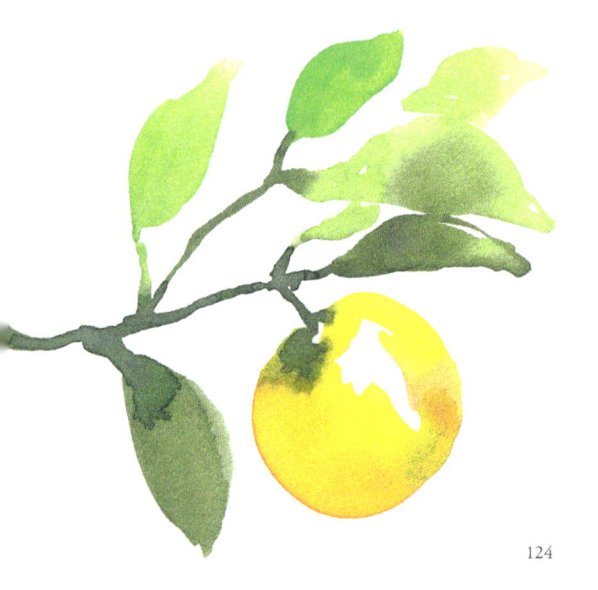

EXERCISE: BEFRIENDING YOUR NERVOUS SYSTEM

Grab a pen and paper.

Think about a challenge (either past or present) and describe it in a few sentences. Write about the thoughts and feelings you experienced during this time and what this might reveal about the state of your nervous system.

As best you can, really identify which aspects of the challenge felt like red zone experiences. (You can refer to the previous list for assistance.)

Write these down.

Reframe this challenge using the non-judgemental language of your nervous system:

My nervous system switches into the red zone when I'm really busy. From this red zone state, I judge myself harshly and ruminate about all the things I didn't get done.

Take three breaths (remember, the long exhale really helps).

Acknowledge that you have moved into the green zone and that your relaxation response has been triggered.

Take a moment to write about this challenge from this more open state.

This might include expanding your perspective, softening the inner judgement, and ruminating or worrying less:

When I notice myself moving into the red zone I can pause, take a few deep breaths, and really come into the present moment. From here, I will feel less self-critical and more realistic about what really needs to be done today.

How to be sensitive and successful

Having a sensitive or highly responsive nervous system or a history of trauma, burnout, or illness, doesn't mean you can't be productive or have big goals and dreams for your future. Take me as an example. Over the last three years, I've created an app, written a book and ten courses, all whilst raising a family, navigating the global pandemic, and healing from chronic pain.

I did this by being mindful of my thoughts, actions, sensations, and motivations whilst in the doing state. Over the years, I have learnt to pause a few times each day and ask myself these questions:

- Is what I am 'doing' right now in line with my values, beliefs and goals?
- Is the motivation behind this activity wholesome? Am I doing it because I *want* to or because I think I *should*?
- How does my body feel?
- What thoughts am I having?

These questions have allowed me to understand my behaviour and become aware of when my actions are triggering my stress response and moving me into the red zone.

For example, I noticed that my nervous system became activated and my stress response switched on when:

- I was performing tasks that I thought I *should* do.
- My inner motivation came from fear of being judged or not accepted.
- I was doing one thing but my mind was thinking about all the other tasks on my to-do list.

In contrast, I also noticed that my nervous system remained in the green zone when:

- I was engaging in tasks that were in line with my values and goals.
- My inner motivation was wholesome, and I was being of service (to family, friends, or the community).
- I was present whilst completing these tasks (my mind wasn't in the past or the future).

Walking the pathway of calm isn't about meditating all day, staring at the clouds, or lying on the couch doing nothing. You don't have to attend a yoga retreat or have years in therapy (although you can if you like). You can explore this happiness avenue anywhere, anytime.

It's about engaging in your everyday activities from a healthy doing state and ensuring your actions are in line with your values and have wholesome motivations (we'll discuss this more in the purpose chapter, I promise). It includes acknowledging when you have moved into the red zone, the trance of busyness, and daring to take the necessary steps to come back to the green zone.

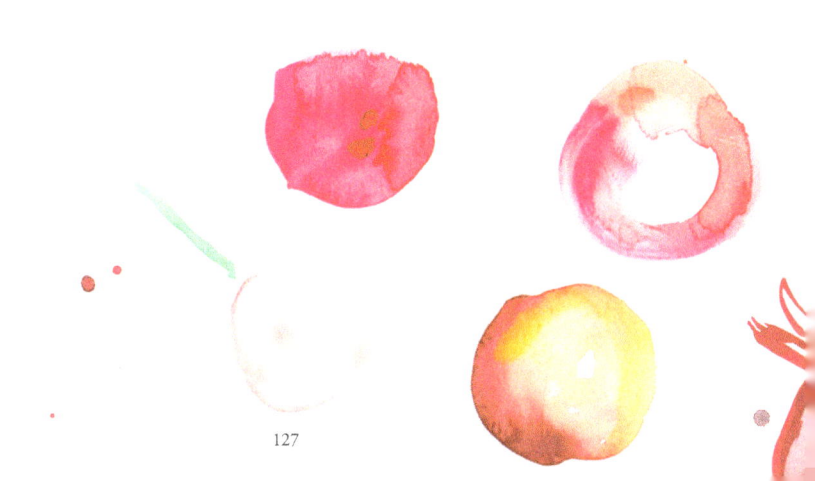

Learning to respond rather than react

Too much time in the red zone can hurt us in many ways. It can create stress within our bodies, encourage highly charged emotions, and cause strain on our relationships. One harmful red zone habit is when we *react* (in haste or autopilot) rather than pause and take the time to *respond* from the green zone.

We've all been here! Maybe you can remember the time you sent that terse work email, raised your voice with the kids, metaphorically rolled your eyes at your parents, or beeped at a stranger in another car.

As a general rule, reacting to life, ourselves, and others from the red zone rarely results in the outcome we desire or allows us to be the best version of ourselves. We usually say something that we later regret, feel ashamed, guilty, or get caught in the self-critical rumination trap. Thoughts like, *I wish I hadn't said that!* flood our awareness.

Amazingly, sometimes the difference between reacting and responding is just a few deep breaths and the power of a pause. That micro-moment where your nervous system shifts gears, your perspective broadens, your emotions feel less charged, and you get to choose the words that come from you. From the green zone, we can have a more balanced conversation and act in greater alignment with our values (for example, love, compassion, or fairness).

EXERCISE: THE POWER OF THE PAUSE

Find somewhere comfortable to sit. Take a few deep breaths.

Cast your mind back to a time when you had an interaction with someone (a family member, friend, colleague, or stranger) and you reacted rather than responded.

Take the time to recall the words, feelings, and body sensations of that moment.

No need to judge yourself or the other person. Remain open and curious.

Now imagine yourself in this moment pausing and taking three deep breaths, really allowing your exhale to feel long and smooth.

Notice your body language and your facial expression change.

Sense into how your emotions feel less strong.

Imagine yourself responding from the green zone.

What would you say or do?

What would they say or do in response to you?

Take a few deep breaths into this moment you have created in your mind.

Trust that this practice will make it easier for you to pause, take a few breaths, and respond rather than react next time!

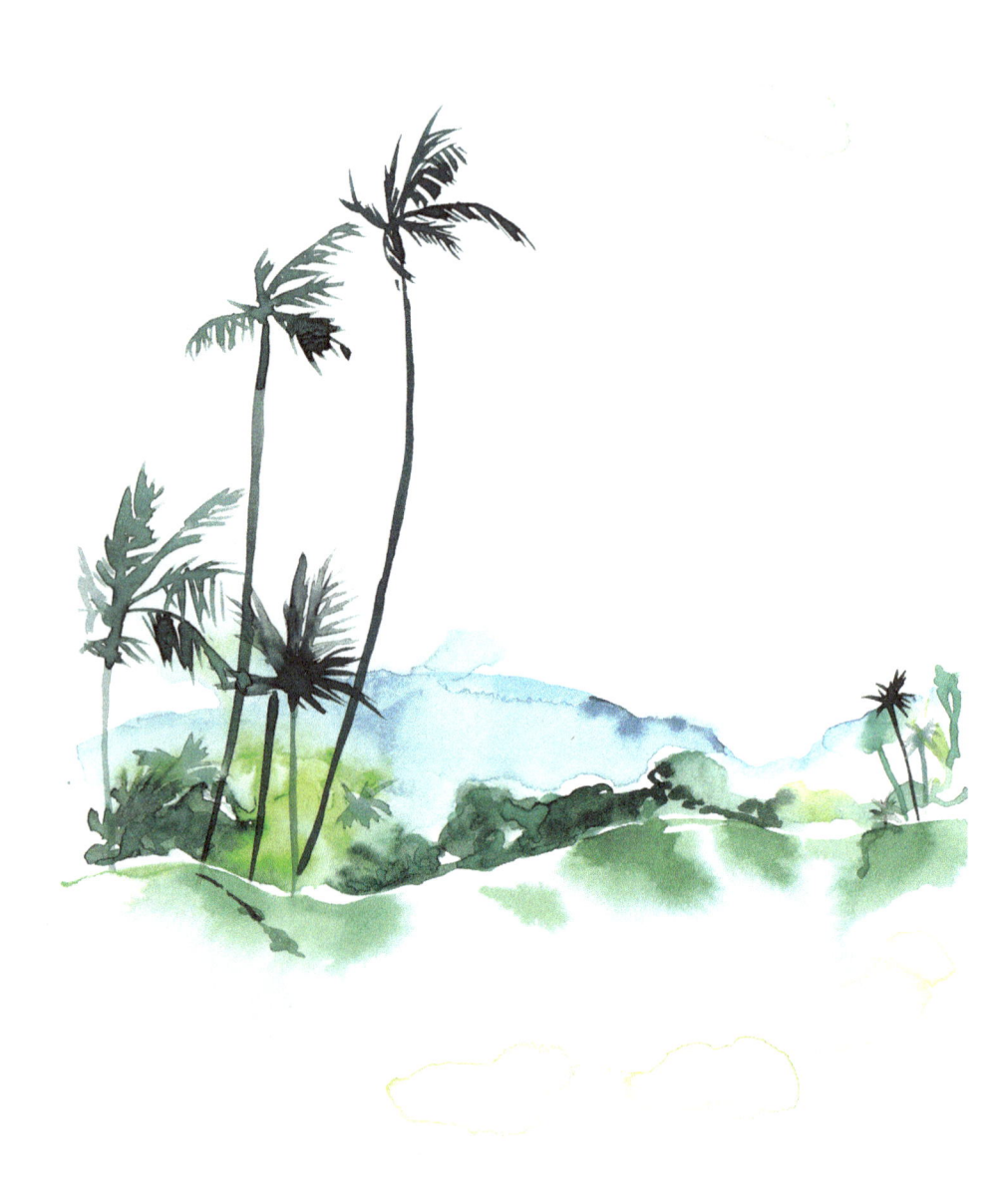

Creating islands of calm in your day

Life is wobbly, messy, and full of setbacks, disappointments, and inconveniences. Delayed trains, bad haircuts, bitter coffee. Uncomfortable conversations with work colleagues, a difference in opinion with someone we like or love. Aging parents, sick children, and financial stress. These challenges, big and small, are part of life. And many of them will engage our stress response.

When we feel agitated, overwhelmed, or like our nervous system is in overdrive, there is nothing more annoying than someone telling us to relax or 'just calm down'. Whilst (sometimes) well-meaning, these comments often serve to agitate us even more. Or, we add something like yoga, meditation, or a walk with a friend, onto our already long to-do list and feel even more overwhelmed.

Rather than 'trying (striving) to relax', a more skilful approach to managing the build-up of stress in our everyday lives is to enjoy the process of learning to 'soothe your nervous system'. When we appreciate and cherish our ability to move from the red to the green and when we see this as a radical act of generosity and self-care, our lives change in profound ways. What a wonderful gift to give your body exactly what it needs!

We can learn to soothe our nervous system by creating 'islands of calm' in our days, these micro-moments when you intentionally shift from the red to the green zone. The good news is you've already practiced some of these in the previous chapters.

Three micro-moments of calm (backed by science, of course).

Self-compassion

When we offer ourselves kindness, care, and understanding, oxytocin and endorphins are released, and we move into the green zone. When you notice yourself rushing, striving, or being self-critical, you can pause and take three deep breaths. Focus on the fresh oxygen landing in your chest (and your heart). You can even place a hand on your chest if you like. Notice any emotions or physical sensations without judgement. Offer yourself a soothing phrase like, *Life feels really hard right now*, or, *I won't always feel this way*. Really allow this micro-moment to bring you back into your body and to remind you that you are your own friend.

Gratitude

When we shift from expectation to appreciation we trigger our relaxation response. When you notice your mind becoming judgemental or blaming (of yourself or others) you can pause and take one deep breath. Then ask yourself this simple question: *What is one thing I can see right now and feel grateful for?* You might notice a tree, a child, your dog, or your fridge. Take a deep and grateful breath. Encourage your body to relax. Trust that you have just moved into the green zone.

Letting go

All the small inconveniences and setbacks in our day can build up and form physical, mental, and emotional stress. Learning to let go is a powerful way to return our bodies, minds and hearts to a state of balance and equilibrium. When you notice your stress levels rising, you can pause and take one deep breath. Then try as best you can to lengthen your exhale. For the next few breaths, count to four on the exhale. Then ask yourself: *What can I let go right now (a past conversation, a regret, a worry, physical tension)?* Imagine this thing leaving your body with each exhale. Trust that you have just hopped off the hamster wheel and can now interact with life from the green zone.

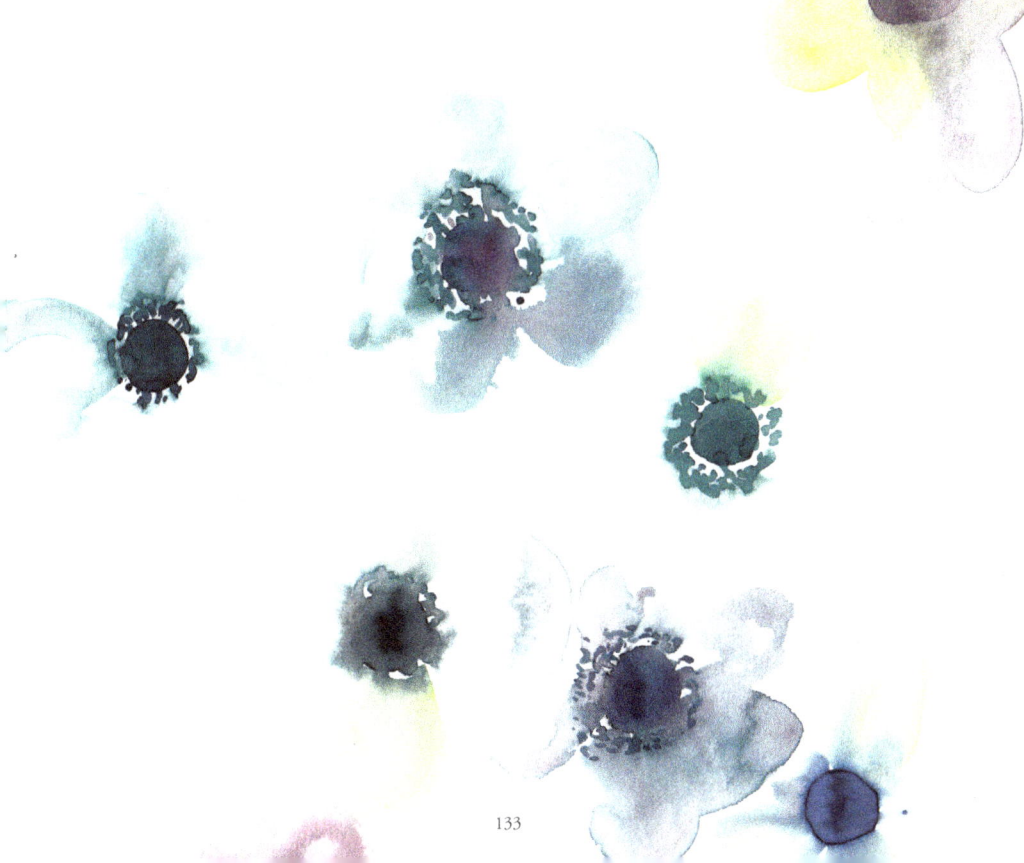

Remember, your body is your first home

My husband has started telling dad jokes ... and it's contagious. I've started telling teacher jokes too. Living in Australia, I'm often a day ahead of my community of meditation students, many of them residing in America and Europe. We typically meet Monday mornings my time, Sunday evening their time. When we meet virtually I love to assure them they have nothing to fear, that the future is bright! The delight I take in sharing this time travel joke never fades.

My joke points to our new reality. We have the capacity to connect with people in all different locations and time zones. We can have breakfast at home and go to bed in another state or even country. Whilst our minds can move from place to place or idea to idea in a flash, our bodies are still human — desperate to have two feet on the ground and to be reminded that they are safe.

Much-loved Australian author, David Malouf, reflects upon our fast-paced lives and the implication for experiencing contentment in his article, 'The Happy Life', featured in *The Quarterly Essay*. He explains, 'We are still bone-heavy creatures tied to the gravitational pull of the Earth.' We must remind ourselves each day that our physical body is our first home. By offering our bodies presence, respect, and gratitude, we feel more content.

EXERCISE: COME HOME TO YOUR BODY

You can try this practice whenever you notice yourself in the unhealthy red zone.

Pause. Take a few deep breaths (long exhale).

Soften the space above your eyes.

Allow some space between your upper and lower teeth.

Encourage your shoulders to drop a little.

Take a deep breath into your chest.

Feel your feet on the ground.

Rub your hands together. Really feel the warmth you have created within your hands.

Place your hands somewhere on your body that feels good for you.

Repeat silently in your mind a few times:

I am safe in my body.

Notice how it feels to come back into your body.

Rest here for five breaths, really allowing your exhale to feel long and smooth.

Repeat silently in your mind:

When I feel safe in my body, I feel safe in the world.

Offer yourself a smile as you've just moved into the green zone, the place where happiness naturally grows.

PATHWAY SIX: CONNECTION

Trust the mystery and wonder of the world

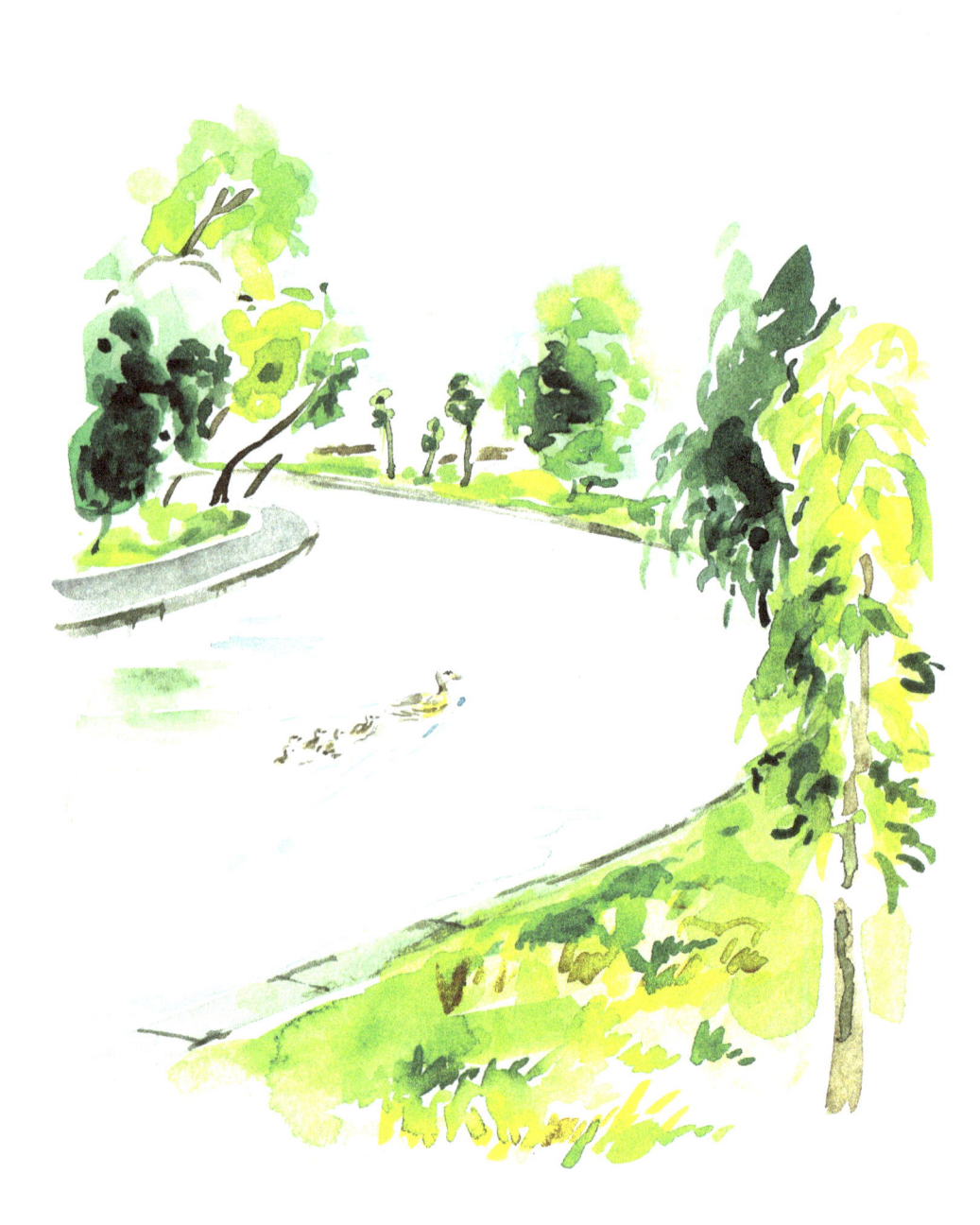

What would your life look and feel like if you learnt to cherish rather than control?

Just as a lightning bolt ignites the night sky, ideas come like a flash of light, instantly awakening something within me. In that moment, I am inspired and ready to take action. Call it intuition, decision-making on steroids, or even haste, it's not important. What matters is that, over the years, I've learnt to listen and trust these ideas more than the voice that often arrives shortly afterwards — the devil of inner doubt, ready to spoil these moments of pure inspiration and clarity.

I knew I wanted to marry my now-husband after only one month of dating. I decided to create a meditation app one morning over peanut butter toast with a friend, having never entertained the idea before. One evening, as I lay in my son's bed as he fell asleep, just like a shooting star across the sky, the idea for this book moved across my awareness.

Each time these big ideas land, I take a grateful breath and say thank you. I feel deep into how privileged I am to live in a country where it's possible for women to have bold ideas, and the resources and support to bring them to life.

Eighteen months ago, in spring, I was walking along the local canal. There wasn't a breath of wind, which was uncharacteristic for that time of year. My gaze landed on a family of ducks — mother duck at the front and three ducklings swimming behind. They had soft fluffy feathers and webbed feet, like tiny paddles, moving beneath the surface. The trail they left on the water was perfect, each ripple like a stroke on a giant canvas. At that moment it came to me, almost as if the words were written in their wake: I want to learn to talk to animals.

Whilst I trusted in this new idea, it also surprised me a little (as you can imagine!). Don't get me wrong, I like animals, but back then, my family and friends wouldn't have described me as 'an animal lover'. I'd never had a chicken coop in my back garden or taken an injured possum to the vet. Every time a bird comes into our home, I pay my kids five dollars to guide the bird calmly back outside whilst I hide under my bed covers. Spiders on my ceiling at night, well, that's my husband's domain.

Despite all this, over the following weeks, I found myself fantasising about travelling to the tropical rainforests of Central Africa to share heartfelt moments with gorillas. I imagined absorbing the ancient wisdom of the powerful condors in flight against the backdrop of the Andes mountain ranges in South America. I created clear visuals of orangutans in Indonesia smiling at me with their eyes and offering me forest wisdom.

I look back on these grand ideas now and laugh quietly at our human tendency to always go for the most exotic expression of our desires. When we are tired and overwhelmed, we fantasise about cocktails by the pool on an imaginary holiday. When we are feeling bored or lacking in direction, we envisage ourselves doing something truly remarkable, like running a marathon, starting a charity, or relocating to the other side of the world.

Then came the global pandemic, when our world shrunk to a 5km radius. This made talking to the gorillas, condors, and orangutans a little challenging (unless I was going to add telepathy to the mix. And as far as I was aware, this wasn't written in the wake left by that sweet family of ducks).

So I got curious and creative. I opened to the more localised ways I could begin to communicate with animals. The answer was simple. It had been there all along. Our family dog, Lucky. I began by opening the lines of communication between me and her. I invited Lucky into my meditation practice. I noticed how her breath deepened as she relaxed and how masterful she was at softening her entire body. When my meditation teacher asked us to sink deeper, Lucky would let out one huge sigh, inviting me to do the same. Sometimes she would make small noises of delight, almost like laughter. I listened. I allowed her to show me that joy is always available.

I listened to the laughing kookaburra perched on the old gum tree down the road with both interest and pleasure. Its perfect song was an invitation for me to lighten up and reconnect with my childlike spirit. I noticed with delight how this iconic Australian bird continued to laugh even whilst my dog barked and barked. Another message to stay in my own lane and not get distracted by the opinions or reactions of others.

When swimming in the sea, I noticed a small and unremarkable fish in my peripheral vision. I knew without doubt that it was urging me to go deeper, both within the water and life. I received its message loud and clear — you have nothing to fear.

I now understand that this calling to 'talk to animals' represented a deeper desire that was growing within me. It was a yearning to connect more fully with nature. It was a tender invitation to trust in the natural flow of life and to believe that I was safe amidst the mystery and the wonder.

We need more green

Perhaps, over recent months, you've had a similar calling. Maybe for you it's presented as an urge to go hiking in the mountains, to swim in the ocean every day, or to ride your bike to work. Perhaps you've committed to finally establishing that veggie patch, taking better care of your indoor plants, or enjoying an evening walk more regularly.

Can you sense into the deeper desire or truth that sits beneath these hobbies or activities? Is there a yearning to break free from your busy thinking mind, the incessant ruminations, the worrying, or the planning? Are you ready to feel less like Sisyphus, the king in Greek mythology, who was forced to push an immense boulder up a hill for eternity? Can you hear the whispers that there is more to life than striving towards a financial or productivity goal?

Is there a part of you that knows that nature and its effortless rhythm may hold the key to a greater sense of ease and contentment? Or perhaps you are ready to feel more alive and grateful for the miracle that is each day on planet Earth?

If you are feeling this longing to spend more time in nature, you are not alone. People from all different life stages and circumstances are feeling it too. All around the world people are embracing the Japanese practice of forest bathing, enjoying a tree or sea change, and ocean swimming all year around. We're choosing to holiday in wi-fi-free zones, build vertical gardens in apartments, sit in the local park at lunchtime, and fill our workspace with indoor plants.

In her book, *Phosphorescence*, Julia Baird offers a detailed review of the research that attempts to better understand the health benefits of spending time in nature. She states that when we are exposed to sunlight, trees, water, or even just a view of

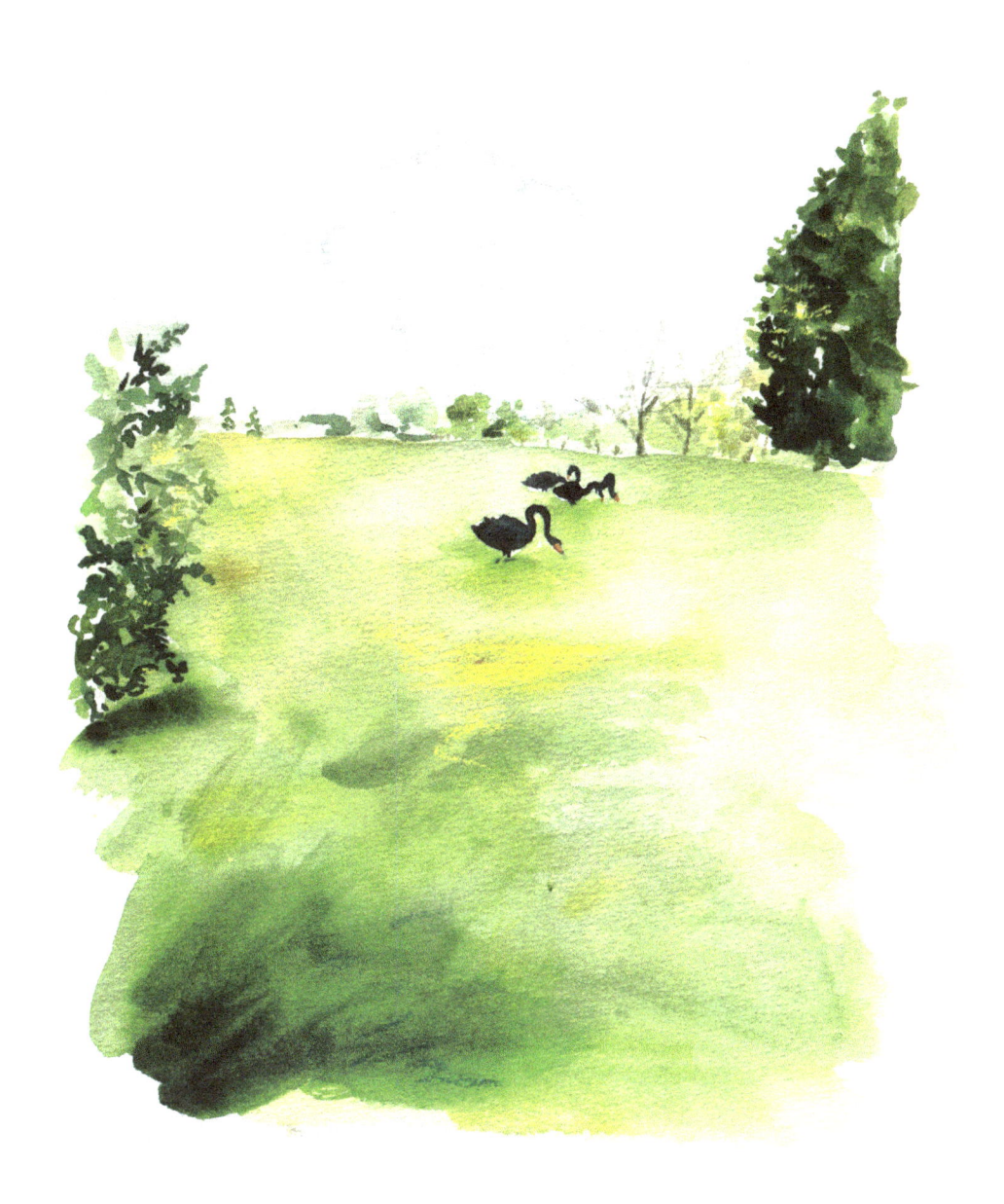

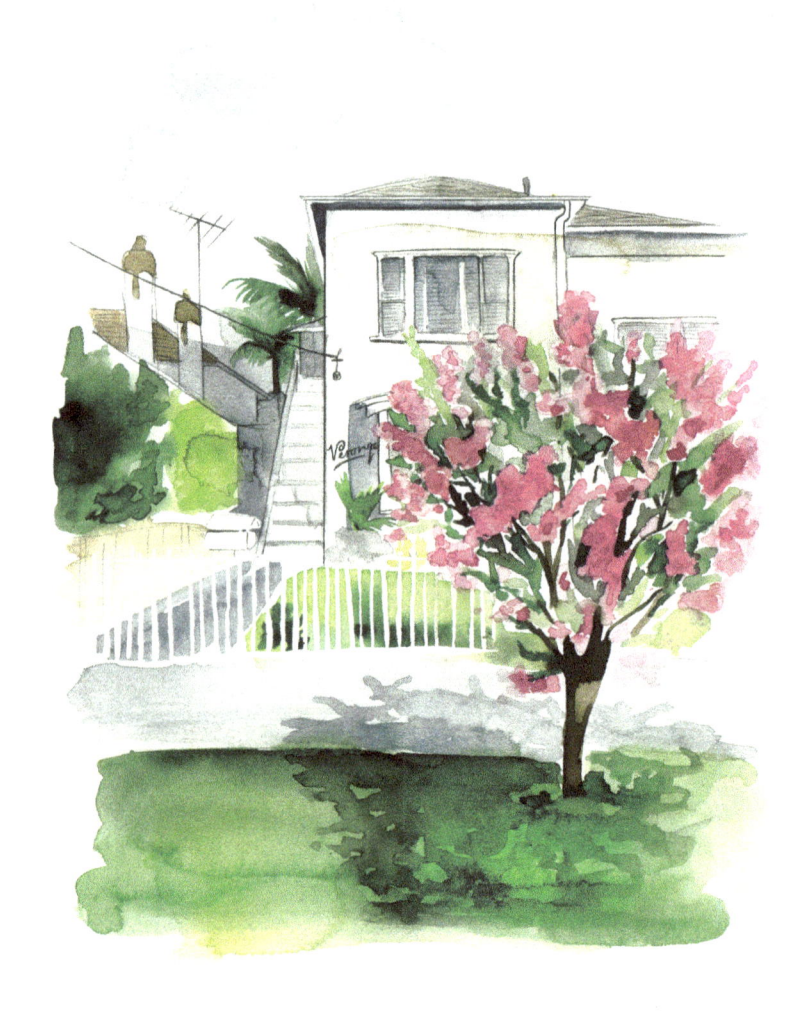

green leaves, we become happier, healthier, and stronger. We have more energy and a greater sense of purpose. Depression lifts, aggression decreases, and concentration improves. Inmates in prison become less physically or mentally ill, hospital patients require less painkillers, and school children perform better in tests.

In 2021, my hometown of Melbourne, Australia, was classified as the most locked-down city in the world during the pandemic. During this period of heightened restriction, many of us experienced firsthand the healing benefits of nature. We used our allocated hour of 'outside time' to take a walk in our local community. We noticed the flowers in our neighbour's garden, the birds, and the signs of the changing seasons. We experienced in real and undeniable ways how small moments in nature calm our anxious minds, relax our tense bodies, and lighten our heavy hearts. During this stressful time in our history, we remembered that just like the sun, we would rise again tomorrow as individuals and as a collective species.

My first mindful year

It's funny how ordinary moments can become forever etched in your mind, and how, with the passing of time, you can begin to understand their significance. I distinctly remember one morning, ten years ago, when I got out of my car and heard the birds chirp. In that moment, a wave of delight washed over me. It felt like their song was just for me.

This lovely feeling was quickly replaced by shock as I realised that I hadn't heard a bird since before my kids were born four years before. I lived in a leafy neighbourhood so I knew birds were there, but in that entire time, I didn't ever notice them.

Could I have been so caught up in my own thoughts, so busy criticising myself for not being a perfect mother or planning the micro-details of tomorrow, that I hadn't been able to hear the delightful song of birds? I was left wondering, *What other sensory wonders had my busy mind been shielding me from?*

At the time, I'd been practicing mindfulness and meditation for a few months. It suddenly dawned on me that this moment of bird song was my reward for daring to break free from the relentless rumination, worry and anticipation that had been consuming me since my kids were born.

This simple moment marked the beginning of my love affair with the sensate world. I began by opening my senses to my family life. The sweet sound of my children's laughter; the feel of their small warm hands in mine; the sight of their little bodies in matching pyjamas. I quickly noticed that when my senses were alive, the ordinary moments began to feel more beautiful.

I expanded my practice to exploring my senses when I was out and about. I noticed the feel of the warm breeze on my skin; the sound of laughter as people walked by; the smell of coffee coming from the local cafe. Life was in high definition. My mind was waking from the trance of distraction. My heart was opening to the fullness of each day. It felt both peaceful and exciting at the same time.

From here, my mindfulness practice grew to incorporate noticing and connecting to the seasons. I allowed the seasons to gently guide me to my own inner rhythms. Over that first mindful year of mine, the seasons were like an old friend offering me wisdom and gently guiding me home in each moment.

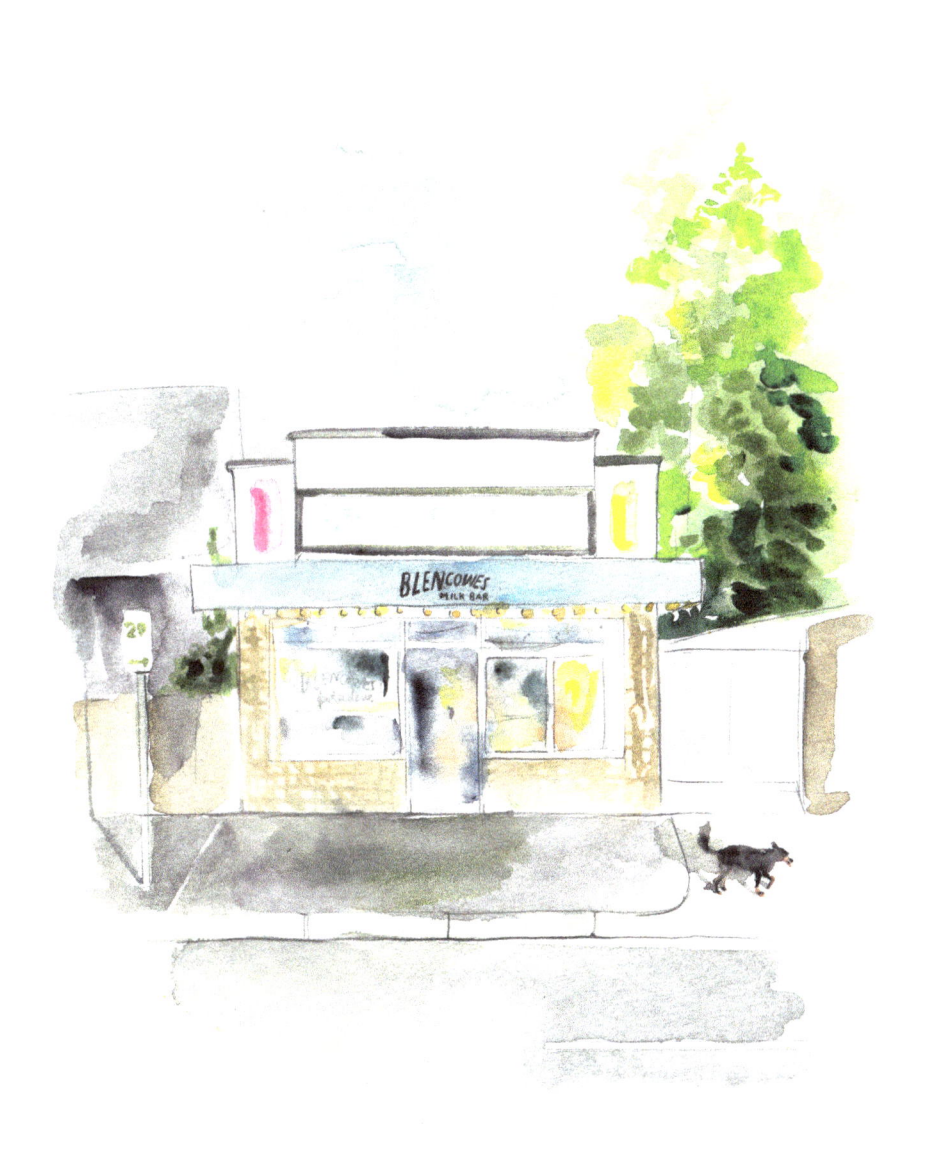

Autumn

As the leaves fell, I explored letting go of the stories, beliefs, and ways of being that no longer served me. I began to soften my need to 'get it right' all the time and instead, welcomed in the natural ups and downs of family life with three small children.

Winter

As the days became shorter and the trees more bare, winter arrived and our life became purposefully more quiet. There was less housework and more meditation. Fewer dinners with five different vegetables and more stories in bed with soft cuddles. Less outer business and more inner peace. I came home to the part of me that was curious, accepting, and compassionate. I enjoyed meeting this less critical version of myself. I know my kids did too.

Spring

The arrival of spring offered me the gift of beginnings, hope, and possibility. I began to birth a new atmosphere within my family, one that included more presence, laughter, and joy. More barefoot ice-cream moments, less battles over bedtime.

Summer

This season came with the message to embrace all life. I began to open to it all, the parts of my life I desperately wanted, and the parts that caught me by surprise. I stopped hurrying through the hard times and wishing away the mistakes. Instead, I began to offer each moment my warm-hearted presence.

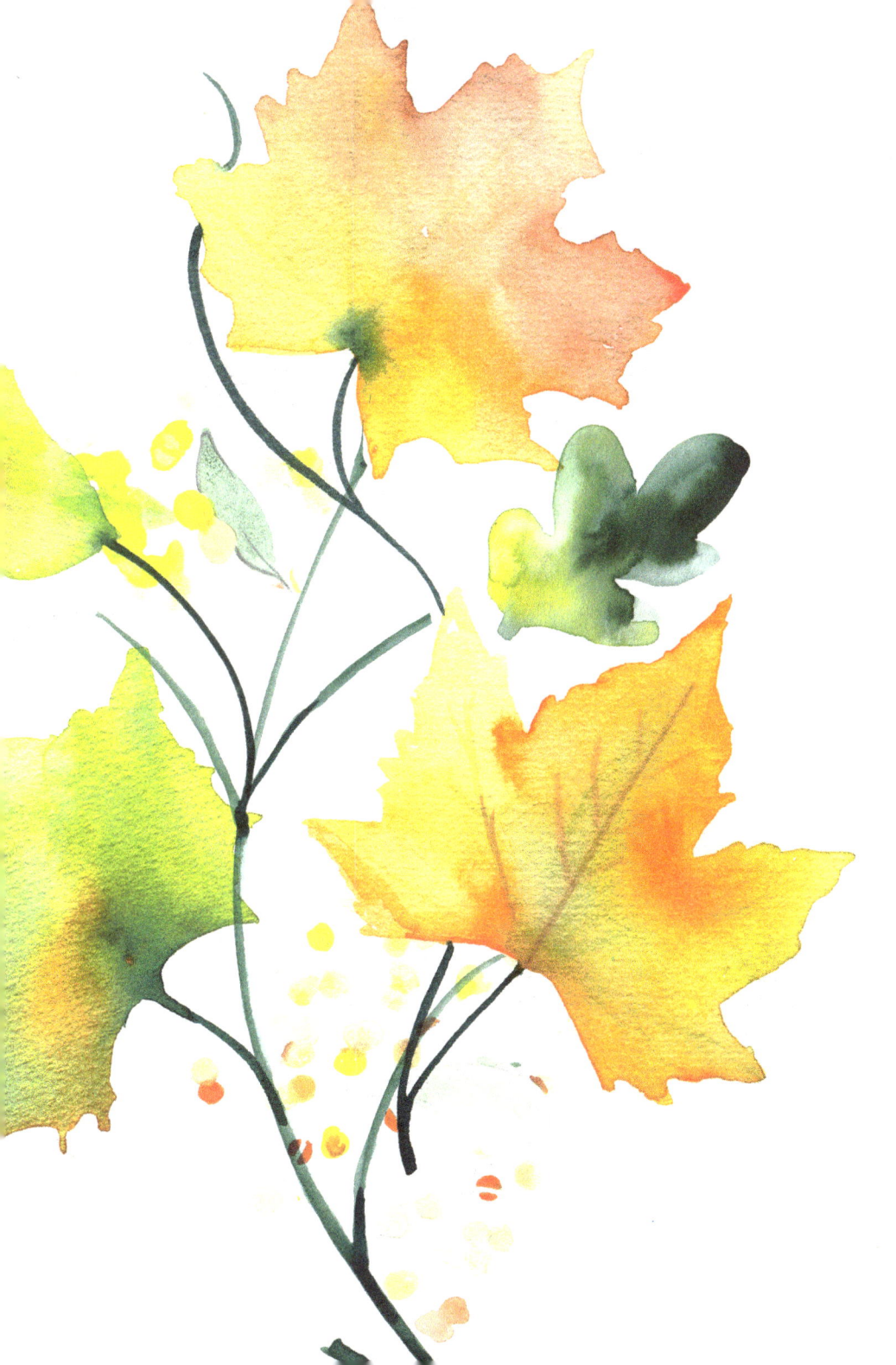

Syncing with the seasons

Throughout history, different cultures have used the seasons to help guide human behaviour, support health and wellbeing, and understand more deeply the human experience. For thousands of years, Aboriginal and Torres Strait Islander People have observed seasonal, meteorological, and astronomical changes. They have followed water, plant, and animal cycles as a way of identifying what to eat and how best to live. Even more than this, they have observed these changes as a way of acknowledging the interconnected nature of life and of deeply respecting and connecting to Country.

The ancient Chinese, Tibetan, and Vedic traditions all invite nature and the seasons to help humans arrive at a state of health and balance. The teachings of traditional Chinese medicine map out five seasons, rather than the four we are used to observing in the West. Each season brings its own energy and its own rhythms that can help us connect with what our bodies need the most. In Tibetan medicine, seasonal knowledge is also regarded as a powerful instrument in the prevention of illness and disease. Since Vedic times, Hindus across India and South Asia have allowed their six seasons to guide their everyday lives and create greater meaning and purpose.

During the time of the Inca Empire, the Pisac Sun Temple served as an astronomical observatory where it was possible to determine the arrival of the solstices and the seasonal changes. It directed the general population when to plant, harvest, and store food. I remember visiting the Sun Temple at Machu Picchu in my early twenties. I hiked in the dark to arrive just as the sun peaked above the horizon line. As the first light shone across this ancient site, I felt touched by the Incas' ability to weave their spiritual beliefs, architectural skills, and knowledge of the sun, moon, and the seasons into their everyday lives.

These examples, whilst diverse, all support the truth that life is cyclical in nature — that it includes creation and destruction, collapse and renewal. The seasons teach us how, in every moment, life is transforming. History whispers to us in both strong and subtle ways that the most harmonious way to live comes from listening, respecting, and receiving the wisdom held within the natural cycles.

In today's world of indoor living, access to heating and cooling systems, and international produce, it's easy to forget about the seasons. So how do you begin to reconnect with their wisdom? Pause and take three deep and intentional breaths. Notice how each breath contains a beginning (inhale) and an ending (exhale). Become aware of how the full cycle of breath is effortless, just as it is in nature.

EXERCISE: SURRENDER INTO YOUR SEASON

Find a comfortable place to sit where you can see nature.

Notice the season you are in. Take in the details of this season.

Sense into what this season represents in nature (for example, beginnings, hope, letting go, or endings).

Relate this season to your own life.

Ask this season:

What lessons do you have for me?

Acknowledge the season that came before.

Acknowledge the season that will come after.

Breathe deep. Rest in the awareness that just like nature, you also have seasons.

Repeat silently in your mind:

Seasons come and go. I am safe to surrender into the natural flow of life.

Nothing lasts forever (and that's okay!)

Have you ever watched your child sleep and felt overcome by a wave of love, only for it to be quickly spoiled by the thought, *They won't always be this small and need me this much*? Perhaps you've been on a holiday and felt relaxed and carefree, only to remember that next week you'll be back at work and the good times will be over? As humans, one of our greatest challenges is to enjoy the moment whilst also knowing that it won't last forever.

This idea of impermanence is an important aspect of Buddhist teaching and one that has filtered into many mindfulness and meditation practices in Western culture today. Impermanence acknowledges that nothing lasts forever. Life, our relationships, experiences, thoughts, and emotions are always changing. When we get attached to certain conditions or situations, when we cling on or grasp, this is when we suffer.

Zen Master Thich Nhat Hanh, the global spiritual leader, poet, and peace activist, described the suffering that is borne from holding on or attaching in his book, *The Heart of the Buddha's Teaching*. He said:

> *'It is not impermanence that makes us suffer. What makes us suffer is wanting things to be permanent when they are not. We need to learn to appreciate the value of impermanence. If we are in good health and are aware of impermanence, we will take good care of ourselves. When we know that the person we love is impermanent, we will cherish our beloved all the more. Impermanence teaches us to respect and value every moment and all the precious things around us and inside of us. When we practice mindfulness of impermanence, we become fresher and more loving.'*

IMPERMANENCE TEACHES US TO RESPECT AND VALUE EVERY MOMENT AND ALL THE PRECIOUS THINGS AROUND US AND INSIDE OF US. WHEN WE PRACTICE MINDFULNESS OF IMPERMANENCE, WE BECOME FRESHER AND MORE LOVING.

THICH NHAT HANH

Impermanence allows us to connect to what is real, not illusion. When we open to the truth that life is always changing, we get closer to the mystery, wonder, and miracle that is each day on planet Earth.

Impermanence invites us to gaze at our sleeping children with love and appreciation, cherishing the moment more deeply as we know it too will pass. It allows us to enjoy our holiday whilst also acknowledging its transient nature. When we allow the energy of impermanence to hold us as gently as one would hold a small child or animal, our hearts open, we soften and experience life more deeply.

Reminding ourselves of the impermanent nature of our experiences can also help us face our challenges in more wise and skilful ways. Take my chronic pain as an example. Whilst the bigger picture is that I've experienced chronic pain for over seven years, when I reflect on the idea that things change, I can see more clearly that my pain hasn't been constant. The sensations have come and gone. My response to it has ebbed and flowed — as have my emotions.

The same can be said for the pain of loneliness, grief, unworthiness, anxiety, or other emotional or mental states. These experiences aren't one-dimensional. They also change. Emotions, thoughts, sensations, and pain all rise and fall. When life feels hard, it can be comforting to remember this truth.

Buddhist monks have dedicated their lives to understanding and embodying these ideas so obviously it's not a practice you will master overnight! As always, begin gently, stay curious, and offer yourself compassion along the way.

EXERCISE: STOP CLINGING, START LIVING

Find yourself a quiet place to sit.

Begin by simply acknowledging that all the things in your environment are impermanent. The couch you sit on, the pictures in frames, the food in your fridge, even your home won't last forever. The people you live with, the relationships you have, the life stage you are currently in, these are all impermanent.

Notice how this awareness makes you feel. Uneasy, grateful, fearful, calm?

Meet whatever arises with compassion. Offer your experience a few deep breaths.

Remind yourself that there is nothing you need to achieve, master, or overcome. Trust that just being here with presence is enough.

Ask yourself these three questions. You may just sit in silence as you reflect on what emerges or you may choose to put your thoughts on paper:

1. How can I use the idea of impermanence to help me feel more grateful for my relationships?

2. What challenge, hardship, or pain can I see through the lens of impermanence as a way of making it feel less overwhelming?

3. What aspect of nature allows me to practice feeling okay with impermanence (flowers in bloom, clouds moving across the sky, the phases of the moon, the path of the sun, falling leaves)?

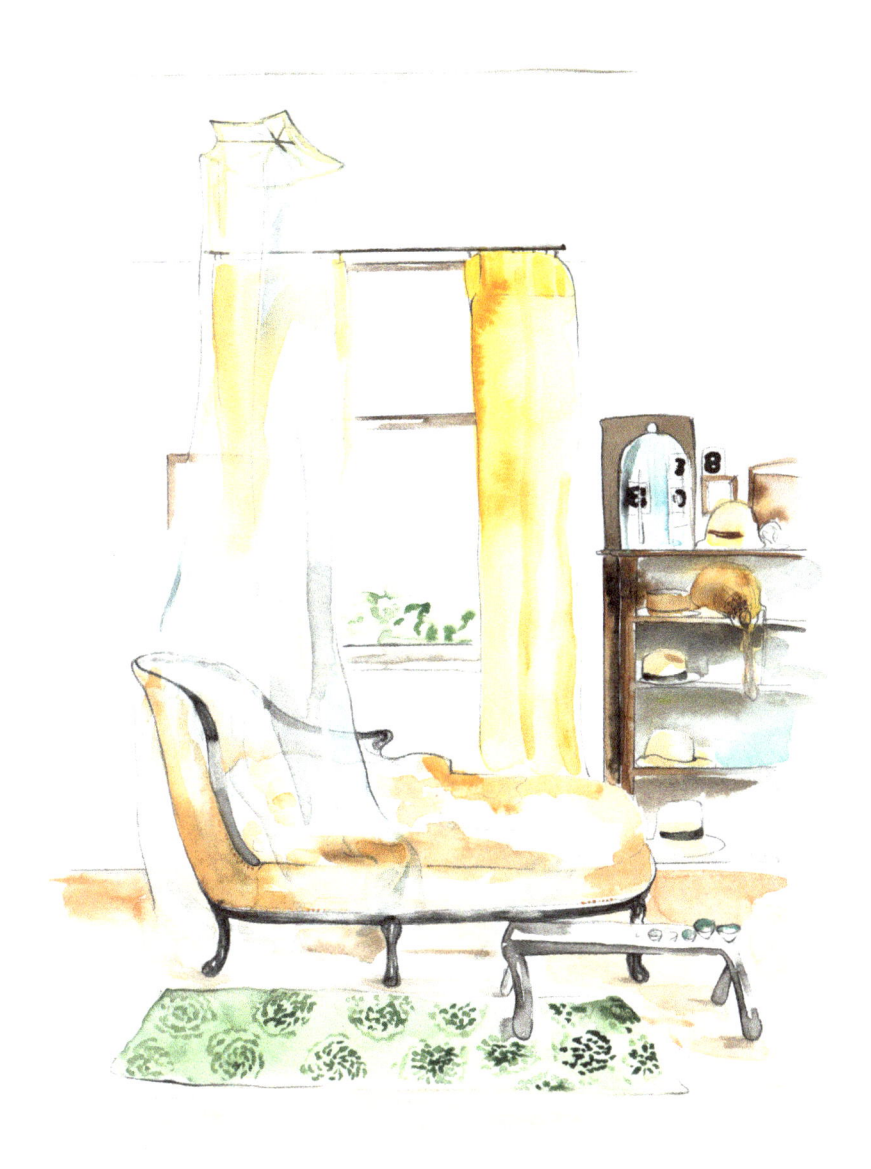

Learning to interact with your life through the lens of impermanence is a radical act. For many of us, it requires relinquishing control (or should I say — perceived control). Trust that when you do (even if for a moment at a time) you'll be more able to appreciate all that you have, your life stage, relationships, and those you love. From here your actions will feel less like clinging on and more like cherishing. I hope you'll notice how the energy of cherishing softens your body, opens your heart and allows you to experience greater happiness. We'll explore impermanence and how it can help us to experience more joy in the vitality chapter too.

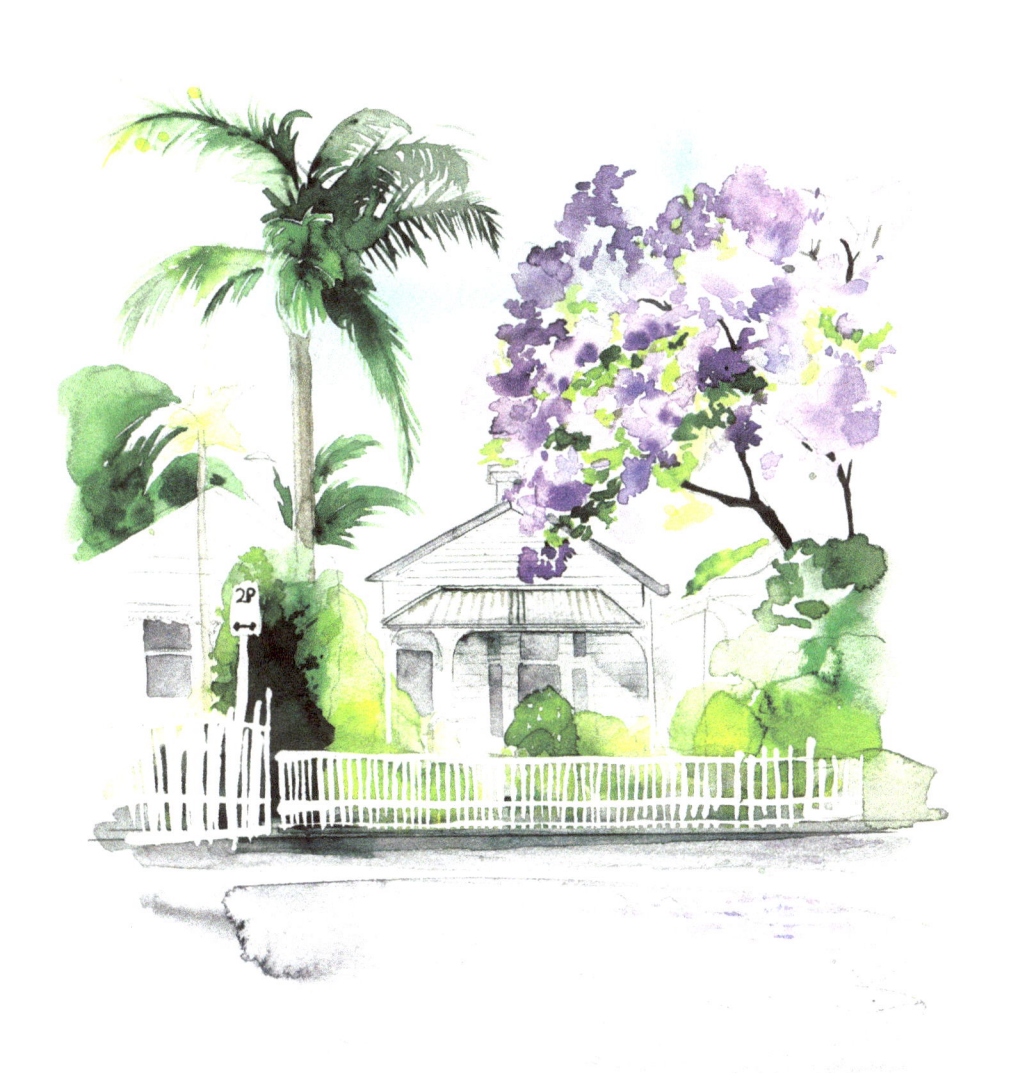

PATHWAY SEVEN: PURPOSE

My life matters, I am part of life

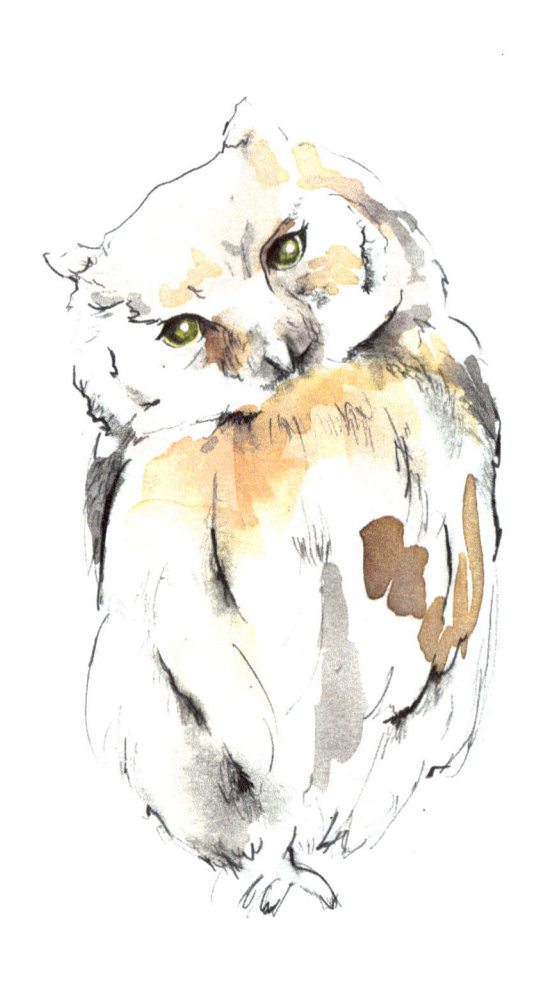

When we notice the synchronicities in our lives, we walk towards greater meaning and happiness.

My husband is physically fit. You don't need to take my word for it — ask anyone who knows us! Every summer, different family members and friends ask him how he keeps in such good shape. I imagine these people hope to discover a magic secret, ideally something fast and free ('I began intermittent fasting three weeks ago and now I look like this').

Instead, he tells the truth, 'I've been exercising four times a week since I was sixteen.' One slow day, I did the maths for fun — that's 6,240 workouts over the last thirty years. In a world of fad fitness trends, I admire my husband's consistency and commitment.

Most mornings he wakes early and lifts weights in the dark on our back deck. I then spend the rest of the day trying not to trip over them. A few months ago during his workout, he was visited by a powerful owl (that's the actual name of the species).

As I was drinking my morning coffee, my husband bounded inside, full of post-exercise endorphins and excitement, eager to tell me about his visitor. The owl had landed on our back fence and sat there, head bobbing, all during his workout.

Whilst I enjoyed witnessing his delight, a thought echoed in my mind, *I'm the one who talks to animals, how come the owl visited him and not me?* (Didn't I mention I'm full of contractions?)

Of course, I didn't spoil the moment by saying those words out loud. Instead, I asked my husband what message the powerful owl had for him. Whilst Andrew is very open-minded and loves learning about scientific discoveries relating to planets and the universe, I wouldn't describe him as 'spiritual'.

To my surprise, he replied without hesitation, 'The powerful owl told me to keep going and to stay strong.' I smiled as I thought to myself, *I guess I'm not the only one in the family who talks to animals!*

Three days later I was making my bed when out of the corner of my eye, something caught my attention. From out my window, I spotted an owl perched on a tree branch. Given its perfect camouflage, it was a miracle I noticed it. A rush of delight washed over me. In my forty-four years, I'd never seen an owl anywhere but the zoo.

I rallied my husband and kids, and we all went outside to take a closer look. The owl blended in perfectly, the mottled grey feathers, the shape of his head, all mimicked the colours and contours of the tree.

My husband was quick to tell me that my new friend was not a powerful owl but a tawny frogmouth. (You see, after his owl encounter a few days before he had done some research on trusty Google and was, apparently, now quite the owl expert.) As we all stood there gazing at this amazing creature, Andrew offered another nugget of wisdom — the tawny frogmouth is not officially an owl as it doesn't have curved talons on its feet.

WE GET CLOSER TO
OUR PURPOSE BY
OPENING TO ALL LIFE.
AT ITS DEEPEST LEVEL,
PURPOSE IS PRESENCE.
THE TYPE OF PRESENCE
THAT FEELS EXPANSIVE,
CREATIVE, FULL OF
POSSIBILITY AND
DELIGHT.

I wasn't going to let this small detail detract from my owl encounter. I thought to myself, *Well, Mr Tawny may not officially be an owl, but he is impressive — powerful in his own way.*

I was hooked. Over the next few weeks, Mr Tawny returned many times. I stood beneath the large tree and enjoyed his company. Given his nocturnal nature, most of the time he was asleep, but every now and then he looked straight into my eyes. In those moments, I felt alive. Something was gently awakening within me — a sense of connection, vitality, and trust.

The tawny frogmouth visited during Melbourne's sixth lockdown when, like everybody in our city (and the world), I was feeling the full weight of the ongoing restrictions. I missed the sense of energy and connection I received from interacting with friends, family, colleagues, and strangers on the street. I longed for that old feeling of optimism and possibility that I'd taken for granted before the pandemic.

I was tired of having to try so damned hard to keep my anxiety at bay. It felt like I was playing a relentless game of tug of war with my mind. It was pulling in the direction of 'worst-case scenario', and I was left, time and time again, pulling it back.

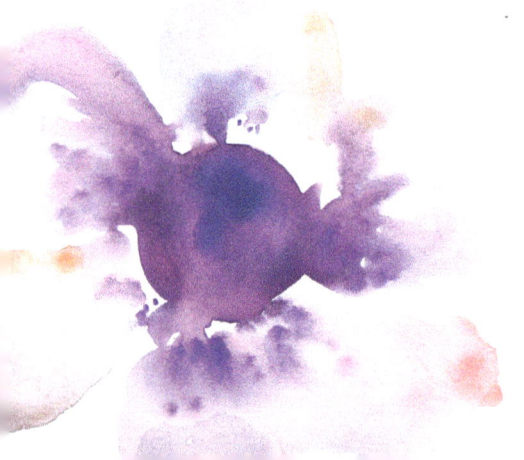

This beautiful bird offered me hope and perspective. It reminded me that there was more to life than the pandemic. Mr Tawny revealed to me that life could still offer us moments of surprise and wonder. Knowing this made me feel lighter and more free. It helped me shift my focus away from fear, towards trust.

A few weeks later, I was in the recording studio creating a twenty-one-day meditation course. I'd written the script a few months before, but due to the ongoing restrictions, it hadn't been possible to record it until now.

The course focused on coming down from our busy thinking minds into the fullness of life. It was about feeling more connected to the natural world, to the mystery and the wonder of life on planet Earth. As I read the script for the guided meditation, a huge wave of emotion and energy rushed over me. I realised that this meditation I'd written a few months back was, in fact, the exact experience I had enjoyed with the tawny frogmouth!

In that moment, the lines between reality, possibility, and mystery blurred like a map left out in the rain. Whilst my logical mind will never fully understand the situation, in that moment, I knew in my heart that all these events were connected. I felt with every cell in my body that I was exactly where I was meant to be, that I was living a purposeful life.

I arrived at the end of the meditation and recited the intention of the practice: 'My life matters, I am part of life.' I smiled and thought to myself — *Yes, indeed*.

Nothing happens in isolation

Has this story allowed you to remember your own encounters with synchronicity? Maybe you can remember a time when you were thinking about a friend and then, at that moment, you received a message or call from them. Perhaps you've experienced the feeling of wanting to take a course or learn something new and the opportunity presented itself with perfect timing.

You don't need to have a spiritual/meditation practice or believe in manifestation to benefit from noticing the synchronicities that life presents you. Opening your eyes to the so-called coincidences, signs, or patterns can alert us to our deeper desires. Like the couple who start trying for a baby and suddenly notice newborn babies everywhere, or the young woman saving for her dream car who now sees them at every stoplight. What about the man who wants to get fit and his friend calls, asking him to join his basketball team? Call it synchronicity, a sign from the universe, or our subconscious bias — all these clues can help us explore our purpose, our desires, and our identity.

Identifying your purpose

So, back to the tawny frogmouth ... It's safe to say that if I'd enrolled in a course on identifying my purpose, I would never have come up with a series of events so mysterious yet true. Can you imagine me in a group Zoom meeting sharing my version of purpose?

I'd say to a bunch of well-intentioned strangers, 'Well, for me, living my purpose will include creating meditations about talking to birds, waiting a few days for a bird to visit me in real life, and then once it has flown away, going into the recording studio to help other people talk to birds too.'

We don't find our purpose by attending a course or using someone else's framework for clarity and direction. We get closer to our purpose by opening to the natural flow and mystery of life. At its deepest level, purpose is presence. The type of presence that feels expansive, creative, and full of possibility.

So, the first step is to stop *chasing* your purpose. It includes letting go of the idea that you should be able to fit your purpose neatly onto a Post-it Note (and if you can't, then your life is devoid of meaning and you are wasting it). The second step is to *trust* that if you commit to being more present in your everyday life, then over time, you'll come to understand what really matters, what lights you up and makes you feel more purposeful.

Ready, steady, flow

No doubt you've heard the term 'in the zone' or even read about the benefits of being in flow (increased performance, heightened enjoyment and creativity, and accelerated learning). But what does the 'flow state' actually feel like? How will you know when you are there?

In his seminal book, *Finding Flow,* Mihaly Csikszentmihalyi, a positive psychologist, explains that flow is 'the holistic sensation that people feel when they act with total involvement'. The flow state, whilst popularised in the 1960s, has roots in Buddhist, Taoist, and Hindu literature.

I like to understand flow as a moment when your mind, body, and heart are all in the same place at the same time.

The flow state arrives like a welcome dinner guest when you are deeply engrossed in what you are doing, when your mind is focused on the activity at hand, your body feels relaxed yet alive, and your heart feels open and receptive.

Ask yourself these simple questions to help you better understand when you are in flow:

- What activities really capture my attention, sometimes making me lose track of time?
- In what situations am I not concerned about how I look or what other people think of me?
- What activities feel like the perfect balance between challenging and rewarding?
- In what situations do I love being part of a group, sharing wins and a collective sense of fun or direction?

Some common activities which may help you feel in flow are swimming, hiking, skiing, snowboarding, team sports or projects, meditation, yoga, dance, cooking, gardening, playing a musical instrument, painting, drawing, or DIY projects.

Flow is a perfect antidote to soothe our distracted minds. Being in flow can be invigorating, inspiring, and fun. It can make you feel alive. Flow can also offer you an experience of peace or serenity. It can help you come home to your deeper nature.

Combining flow with acts of service

For flow to contribute to your sense of purpose, it most likely needs to be more than a game of paintball or soccer with your friends — more meaningful than the momentary endorphin rush after a Zumba or spin class. When our flow activities also include 'being of service', our lives feel more meaningful and rewarding.

We often think that being of service needs to have a Mother Theresa energy, requiring us to be overly kind or compassionate, to work in the health sector or to volunteer our time at an animal shelter or soup kitchen. In truth, there are many ways you can be of service (both directly and indirectly).

I like to use the metaphor of dropping a stone into the middle of a still lake. Just as this one stone creates ripples across the entire lake, your actions can cast positive ripples across your family, local or wider community.

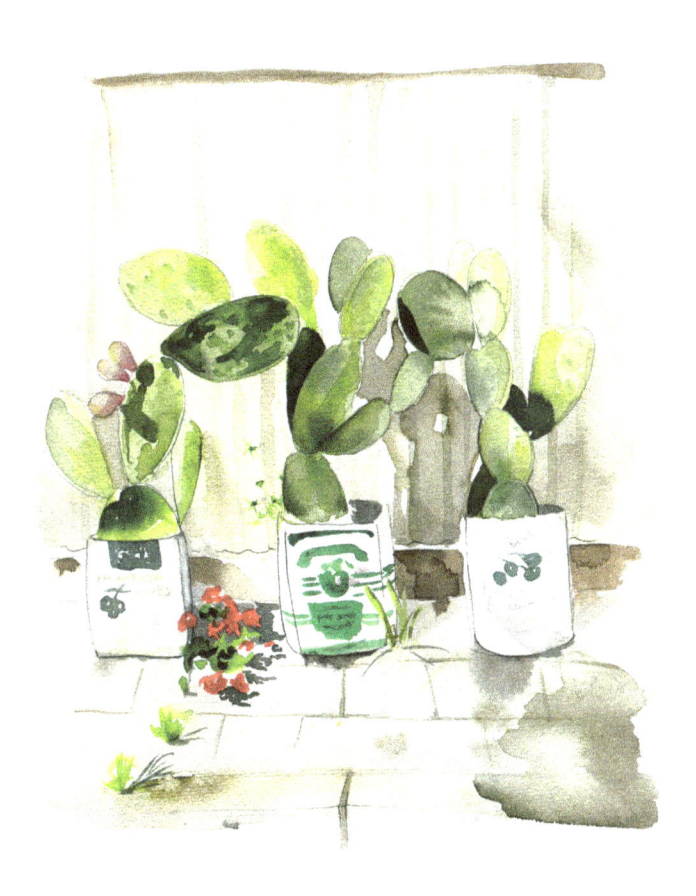

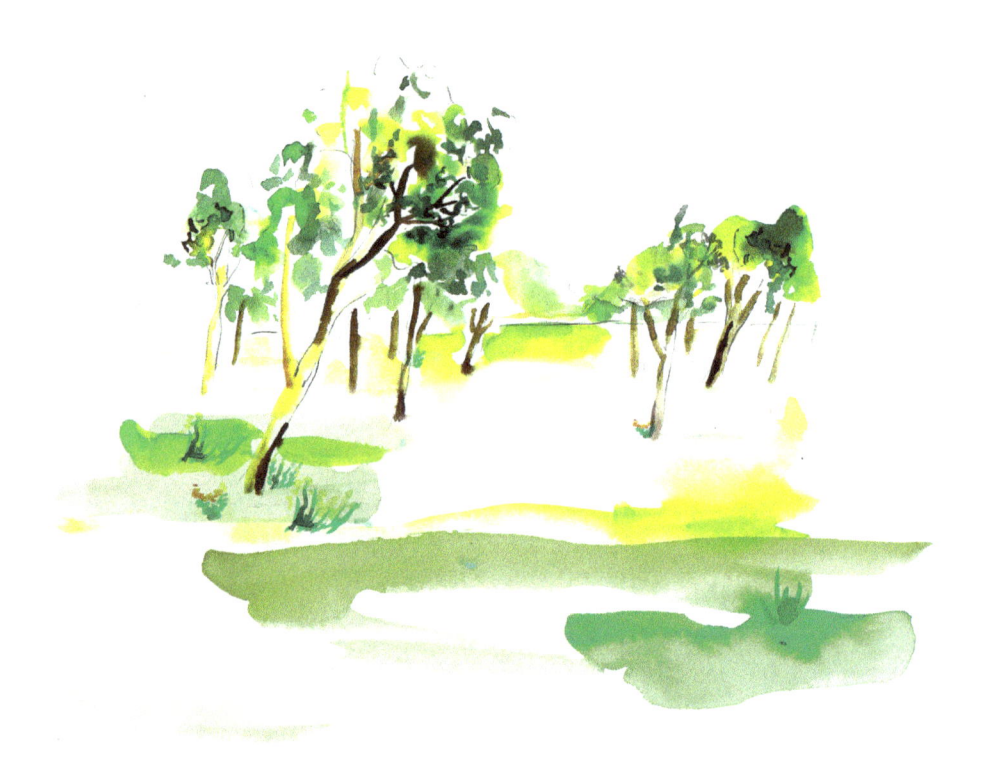

Perhaps you are a teacher or educator and you can imagine all the ways your students will contribute to the world. Maybe you are a parent or grandparent and can reflect upon the impact you are having on your child or grandchild's life. Do you create art, poetry, songs, courses, products, or services that help other people? Do you take delight in cooking for family and friends, or tending to your front garden for passers-by to enjoy?

Ask yourself these questions to help understand how your flow activities may be of service to others or the world:

Does this flow state activity ...

- Support my family, friends, or wider community?
- Contribute to the environment or the positive advancement of our species?
- Support young people or the next generation?
- Help people experiencing illness, disadvantage, mental health, or socio-economic problems?
- Promote creativity, connection, healing, innovation, inclusion, or diversity?

(Please note this is just a guide to get you thinking. It is not an exhaustive list. There are so many ways you can be of service in the world! Trust yourself.)

FLOW + SERVICE = PURPOSE

Grab a pen and paper.

At the top of your page write the two headings: Flow and Service.

Set your timer for three minutes and write down all the activities that provide you with a sense of flow. Remember, these activities can be anything you like and don't need to feel especially wholesome or pure. No guilt here!

Aim for at least ten things on your list.

Set your timer for another three minutes and complete the Service column.

(Get creative as you imagine all the ways that you completing this flow state activity may contribute to the world. Remember the stone in the lake metaphor.)

Read over the list. Identify which activities feel most purposeful.

Write down an intention or goal for how you will do this activity, or ones like this one, more often in your everyday life.

Well done. You just took a big step forward on the pathway of purpose.

Choosing love over fear

In my grandma's last days, she offered me these words, 'In the end, life comes down to two things: love and fear. We must be brave enough to choose love each day.' Over the years, these words have transformed into a regular practice of mine, one that reminds me of her love and guides me towards greater purpose and meaning.

My practice is simple. I pause a few times a day and ask myself two questions:

> What energy is holding me in this moment?
> AND
> What would moving in the direction of love look and feel like for me right now?

For these simple questions to provide insight and direction, we need to become aware of the many ways fear and love can express themselves in our bodies, minds, and hearts. Most of us are familiar with the extreme expressions of fear. We know what a pounding heart, a tight gut, or shortness of breath feel like. We know what anxious thoughts are and what grief, loss, worry, or sadness feel like.

The reality is fear can be more subtle and sometimes even sneaky. It can wear many disguises:

- Judgement towards strangers, family, friends, or ourselves.
- A loud inner critic.
- The desire to blame.
- Repetitive thinking habits such as ruminating, worrying, planning, or strategising.

- Micromanaging the people in our lives.
- Trying to control our relationships.
- Getting pulled in by habits of perfectionism.
- People-pleasing.
- Procrastination.

All the above can carry the energy of fear when we do them.

Love also expresses itself in a variety of different ways. Love is holding us when we:

- Experience a rush of joy or gratitude.
- Enjoy the company of family and friends.
- Are being creative or in flow.
- Enjoy time in nature.
- Dare to be vulnerable.
- Offer ourselves or others compassion or forgiveness.
- Trust that life is working for not against us.

We can all benefit from becoming aware of our unique expressions of fear and love. When we learn to recognise our subtle expressions of fear we can respond before the experience escalates or becomes all consuming. When we notice the gentle signs of love, we can pause, take a breath, become really present, and let the moment land.

YOUR INNER COMPASS (PART ONE)

Try this practice when you are feeling overwhelmed, lost, or unclear about how to move forward.

Begin by taking three deep breaths.

Scan your body. Notice places that feel tight, heavy, or tense. As you breathe, see if you can soften or relax these parts of you.

Acknowledge how you are feeling right now. Notice any subtle expressions of fear. (For example: a loud inner critic, a long to-do list, feelings of worry, overwhelm, or anxiety.)

As best you can, allow whatever is here to be. You don't need to push it away. But also, you don't need to get pulled in. Just breathe.

Imagine you are holding a compass that has two directions, fear and love. In your own time, move the compass so that it points you in the direction of love.

Ask yourself these three questions:

1. What thoughts would help me move in the direction of love?
2. What would be the first action I would take?
3. What do I need to let go of in order to move in this direction?

Really imagine yourself thinking and acting in this way.

Take a deep breath. Smile. You are ready to move in the direction of love today.

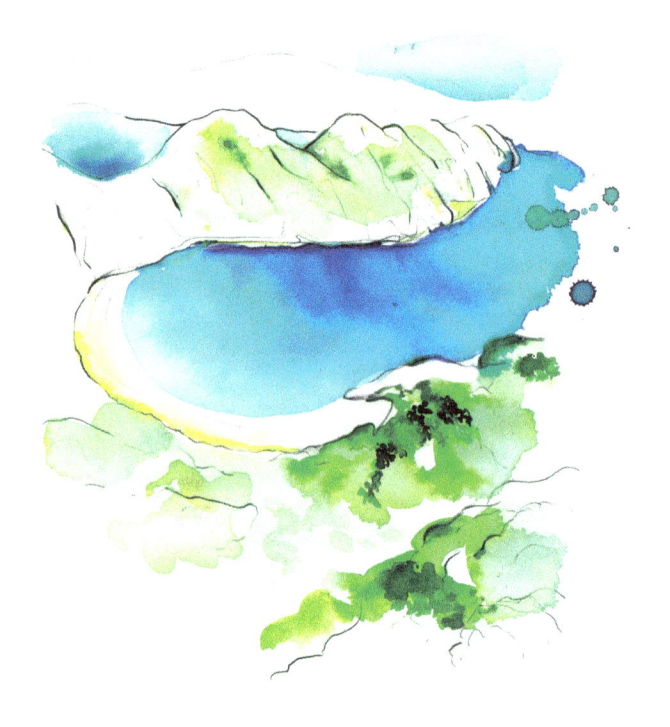

Remember yourself as a child

I grew up near a wild expanse of ocean. When the wind and tide were just right, we would swim amidst the waves, enjoying the thrill of being tossed about. More than just fun, this large stretch of ocean, travelling as far as my little eyes could see, was also a source of great mystery to me.

Over the years, I developed a practice of sitting, watching the ocean, its mood and rhythm, with a deep feeling of awe and appreciation. I would repeat these words silently in my mind: *May the power of the ocean fill me with courage.* This was the eighties, well before the practice of setting intentions became popular in Australia, but there I was, ten years old, sitting in my own prayer with nature.

My secret rituals didn't stop there. As a child, every time I heard an ambulance, I would stop whatever game I was playing and repeat silently in my mind: *May the person in the ambulance, and their family, be okay.* I would imagine sending my love to this ambulance and it sinking into the person who was inside.

Internationally recognised neuroscientist, Dr Rick Hanson, often talks about the importance of staying true to your childhood dreams and inclinations as a way of cultivating wellbeing as an adult. On his podcast, *Being Well*, he explains, 'Our childhood dreams can be like signposts, a guiding North Star that we can come back to as a way to help organise and direct the life we have today.'

So, what clues do these childhood reflections offer me? Do I need to become a professional surfer or a paramedic if I want my life to have meaning? No! But spending time in nature, allowing its wisdom to both soothe and enliven me, would certainly help (and as you heard in our previous chapter, time and time again, I've found healing in nature as an adult).

Practicing compassion, both for myself, others, and the planet is another way I can honour the psyche of my younger self. Finally, these childhood insights illuminate the importance of creating rituals and incorporating prayer into my everyday adult life. Simple things like watching the sunset and thanking it for another day or bringing to mind three things I'm grateful for each morning, are regular practices that offer me comfort. Each time I do these things, I offer the younger version of me a smile, for showing me how to be happy.

EXERCISE: CHILDHOOD DELIGHTS (FOR BUSY ADULTS)

Take a moment to breathe deeply and come into your body.

Notice that your body knows exactly how to breathe. All you need to do is pay attention to the steady rise and fall of your chest and the soft expansion and contraction of your belly.

Take a moment to reflect on the things you enjoyed doing as a child. In a gentle way, open to any memories that emerge.

Really take in the small details of these memories. Notice who was there and what you were doing. Was it day or night? Were you inside or outside?

Notice any emotions you experienced at the time. Were you happy, peaceful, content, filled with joy, excitement, or laughter?

Really allow this memory to provide you with clues about what you love and who you really are.

Ask yourself:

How can I bring more of these childlike qualities into my everyday adult life?

Listen.

Offer this younger version of you a smile for helping you see what really matters to you.

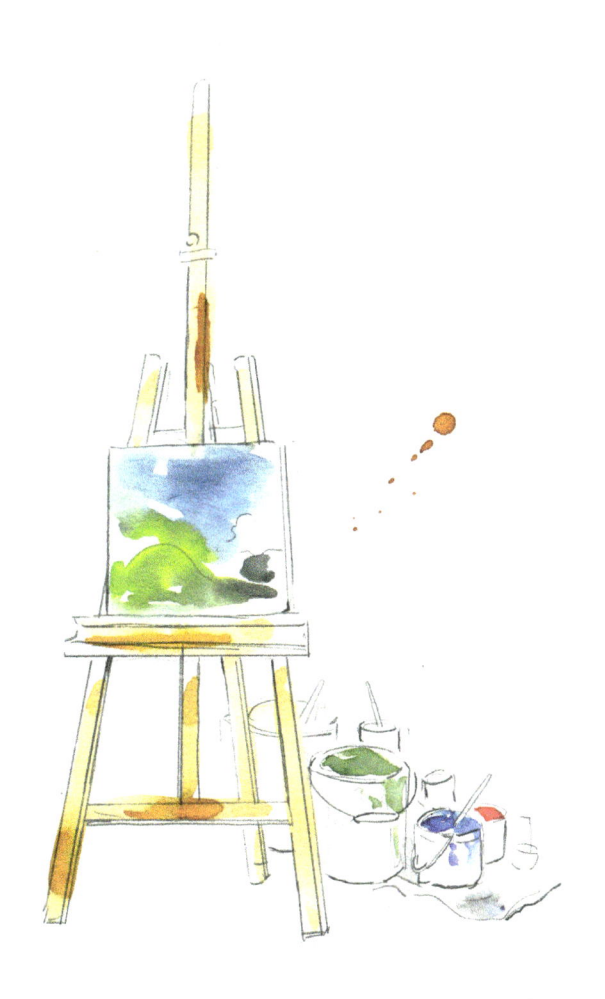

PATHWAY EIGHT: VITALITY

Beyond coincidence to contribution

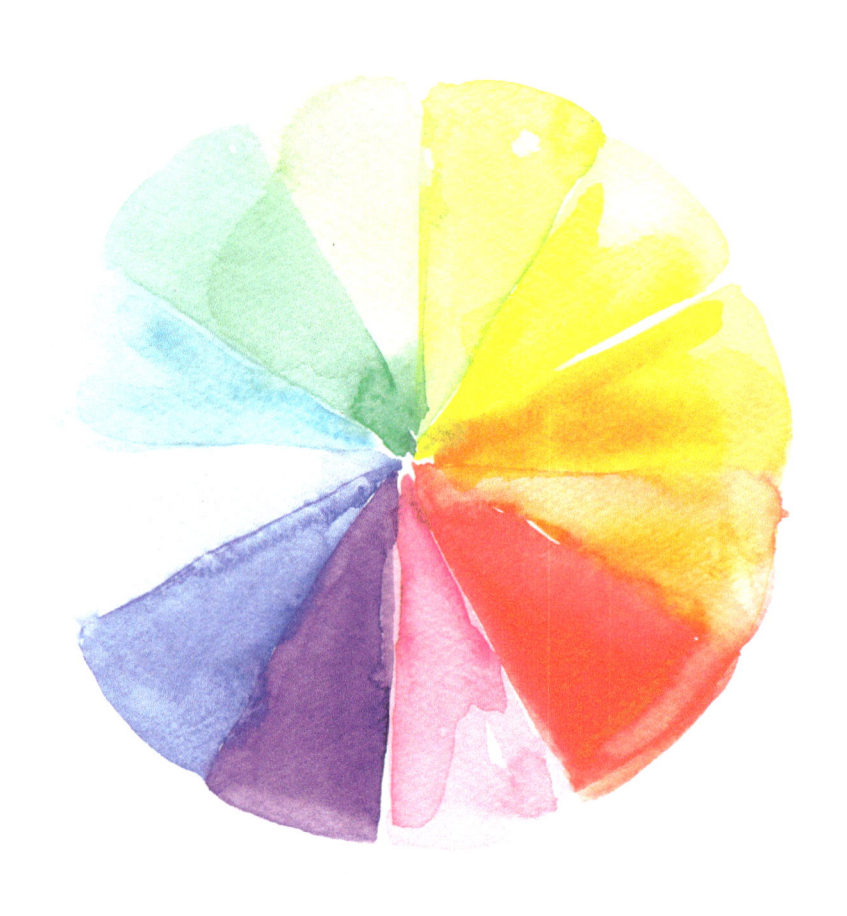

If you want to feel more alive, pay attention to the opportunities to contribute to the world and feel joyful.

Part of walking towards a more relevant and meaningful version of happiness includes a willingness to broaden our definition of vitality. According to the dictionary, vitality is 'the state of being strong and active; energy'.

Social media, advertising, and even the so-called wellness industry send us messages that in order to feel vital and healthy, we should be doing handstands on the beach, taking a selfie on top of a mountain, or completing a triathlon as we hit middle age. Whilst there is nothing wrong with aspiring to be physically healthy, this 'fit and able-bodied' version of vitality excludes billions of people around the world. For example, those who live with major and minor physical disabilities, chronic pain, long-term illness, or the aging population. Don't we all deserve to feel vital?

In order to make this powerful happiness pathway — vitality — more accessible, we need a new definition that relies less on our physical agility and more on our ability to feel connected to life. The best part — this version of vitality can stand the test of time, including injury, illness, getting older, and life's setbacks.

For me, a key to embracing this new version of vitality has been learning to pay attention to the synchronicities around me — the recurring themes that appear in our lives. Some people prefer to call these coincidences, but it's really the same thing — events or experiences in our lives that link together. Like when you want to try something new, and the opportunity magically presents itself. Or like I mentioned in the purpose chapter, when you are thinking about a friend from your past and then they contact you.

These small moments act as reminders that you are on the right track and that your life has purpose. When we take the time to really 'feel' these moments, we experience vitality. For me, I experience a burst of energy inside of me; I know in that moment that life is working for me, not against me. I pause, take a deep and grateful breath, and remind myself that life is holding me, and that I am safe in the mystery (do you notice how I'm letting the moment of vitality land?).

Early experiences, future purpose

Many meditation teachers travel to India, and upon return, speak of a kind of inner transformation. They share stories of connecting to the spiritual power of the Ganges River and participating in religious ceremonies that alter the way they see the world (and themselves). My India experience was a little different.

It was 1985. I was a little blonde-haired, blue-eyed, eight-year-old girl. I travelled with my family from Australia. At the time, it wasn't your typical holiday destination! My parents had a keen sense of adventure and enjoyed learning about different cultures. They had travelled to India before and loved it, so this time they decided to take us three kids too.

We trekked on horseback across the Himalayas. One horse carried a wooden cage containing twelve chickens. Every night, as we set up camp, the chickens were let free to roam. Sometimes my brother (who was ten years old at the time) was given the nearly impossible task of catching the chickens and returning them to the cage. My brother and I couldn't work out why every morning there was one less chicken. Our little minds couldn't (or didn't want to) make the connection to the previous night's dinner!

As we rode the horses who skilfully traversed the Himalayan terrain, we passed different local communities who were living a nomadic pastoral life. Growing up in middle-class suburbia, I had never seen people live in this way. My parents took a photo of me with a group of local children (this photo stayed on our family pinboard for the next twenty-five years).

As I grew up, I would often pause, look at that photo and wonder: *What type of life would these kids have had?* As I completed my various university degrees, I wondered about their education and if they ever had the opportunity to go to school. As I got married and had children, I wondered if they had children and if they were healthy.

These questions often got me thinking about the lottery that is our 'place of birth'. Where we are born and the family we are born into has a huge impact on our lives. In the Western world, it's so easy to assign our successes to hard work, determination, and perseverance without fully acknowledging the incredible start we had by being born into a free and stable country.

An important aspect of my meditation business is supporting international grassroots projects that tackle poverty in some of the poorest communities in the world. Every course or project I create gives back. Over the years, I've provided funding for clean water and mosquito nets in Kenya, counselling for women fleeing domestic violence in Vietnam, solar ovens in Mexico, child care in Burundi, menstrual hygiene in Tanzania, maternal education in Bangladesh, and various COVID-19 related projects.

Finding projects that are aligned with the intention of my work is both exciting and rewarding. It makes me feel vibrant and alive knowing that I can use my teaching as a tool for connecting and supporting people all across the globe, no handstands necessary!

I don't chase these projects, they always find me (here's the synchronicity!). Whenever I'm ready for a new project or a new challenge, a sign comes my way. As I was writing this chapter, it happened again when I met an incredible couple, Bushra and Mushfiq (a microbiologist and engineer), who oversee a 'school in the clouds' in Thanchi, a beautiful and remote part of Bangladesh.

This school sits over 1,000m above sea level and is run by a Buddhist monk for the children who live in these mountains. Each student travels six to twelve hours to get to school and stays for the whole term. When COVID-19 hit, the school was forced to close, and the children were sent into manual labour to support their families. Now, they want to reopen the school, but they would need financial assistance to do it.

As I heard their vision of reopening the school, a wave of emotion and vitality washed over me. I knew without a doubt that this 'school in the clouds' was the project I would support through a portion of the sales of this book.

When I saw a picture of the children who would attend the school, it took me straight back to that photo of me and the Indian children all those years ago. I knew that life was providing me with an opportunity to contribute and feel alive by connecting the dots between my past and present — between the children in India and Bangladesh.

Being aware of what matters to us, noticing synchronicities, and using these as signposts to guide our actions helps us feel vital and alive. You don't need to train for a triathlon, master a handstand, or donate money. Instead, your unique expression of vitality might look more like:

- Allowing the dreams and joys from your childhood to have a place in your adult life (for example: painting, drawing, acting, or reading).
- Acknowledging your interests as a young adult and being creative about bringing these into your later life (for example: travel, politics, sport, or music).
- Sharing your values and what lights you up with family, friends, or your community (for example: being a sports coach, teaching someone to cook, or joining a book club).

Much like purpose, walking the pathway of vitality allows us to remember that life is not happening to us, but rather, that we are part of life. It's a tender reminder that through our awareness and our actions, we can contribute to the world in positive ways.

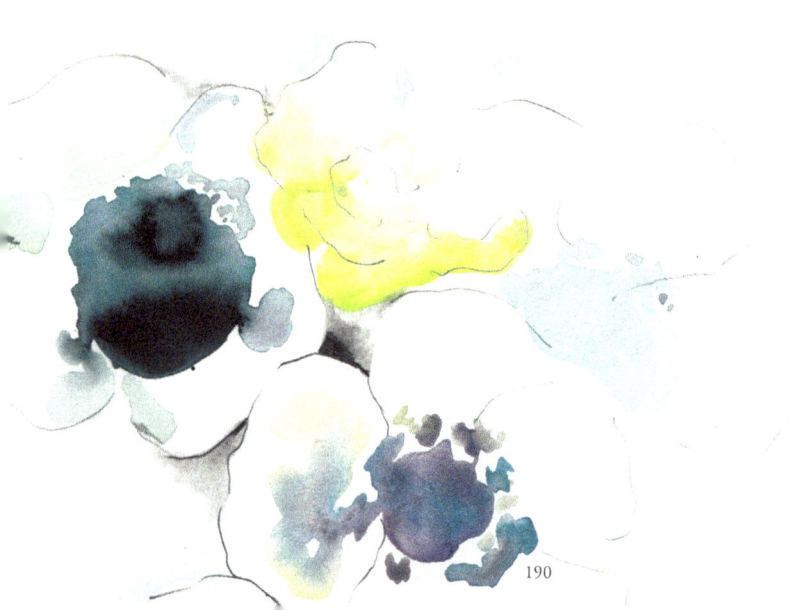

EXERCISE: ACKNOWLEDGING OUR PRIVILEGE

Pause a moment to consider:

As a child, did you assume that all children around the world attended school?

How easily can you access transport? Perhaps you own a car, bike, or scooter. Maybe you can take a bus or train where you need to go. Is this the case for everyone?

The choices you had today in terms of what you would eat and when you would eat.

Your access to medical treatment if and when you need it.

The freedom you have to express your opinions.

The purpose of reflecting on these aspects of our lives is not to elicit guilt or to feel 'pity' for the large populations of people who do not have such opportunities. It's about learning to place our lives in a much larger container of awareness. When we do, we feel more grateful for all that we have and are also more likely to seek out opportunities to contribute to the world. From here, we feel more connected and vital.

Everyday moments packed with meaning

When we move through our days on autopilot, hurrying through one task so we can get to the next, it's easy for the ordinary moments to feel 'vanilla'. Activities like cooking, making the bed, attending to our garden, reading to our children, or taking the dog for a walk can feel like stepping stones — things we *must do* in order to get to the more exciting aspects of our lives.

A key component to feeling more vital is learning to make these ordinary moments feel extraordinary (or at the least, enjoyable!). The first step is completing these tasks mindfully. As we learnt in the awareness chapter, distraction reduces our enjoyment whilst being present, and engaging our senses heightens our satisfaction. The second step includes seeing these everyday moments in a larger context — in particular, in the context of our family of origin.

Before we do this, let me acknowledge that not everyone will want, or be able to, reflect on their family or origin. Some family relationships are unknown, some may be strained or traumatic. In that case, I'm not encouraging you to count your blessings or revisit distressing memories. You can also try this exercise with the support of a mental health expert, therapist, or counsellor.

Begin by taking a moment to consider that for you to be born you needed:

> Two parents.
> Four grandparents.
> Eight great-grandparents.
> Sixteen second-great-grandparents.
> Thirty-two third-great-grandparents.
> Sixty-four fourth-great-grandparents.

Of course, with the increase in reproductive technology and the emergence of more diverse family structures, these figures may not be entirely accurate for you. But I hope you can feel into the basic premise — that you are supported by a long line of family connections.

Imagine all the struggles your ancestors have faced, all the pain and adversity. Imagine also all the moments of love, joy, and happiness. Your ancestors, their lives, their strength, their joy, even their habits are contained in your DNA.

In his book, *Present Moment, Wonderful Moment,* Zen Master Thich Nhat Hanh explained,

> *'If you look deeply into the palms of your hands, you will see your parents and all generations of your ancestors. All of them are alive in this moment. Each is present in your body. You are the continuation of each of these people.'*

When we allow our everyday actions, habits, and hobbies to remind us of those who came before, our lives feel more vibrant. It can also help us feel less alone. Our family (both past and present) don't need to be perfect in order to offer us a sense of connection and vitality. Nor do we need to know these people by name.

I think about these family links every time I hear myself give advice to my kids, which my dad gave to me ('How do you eat an elephant? Piece by piece!'). Or when I feel happy to have bumped into a friend whilst grocery shopping and I'm reminded of how my grandma loved these chance encounters and would always say, 'What a pleasant surprise!' Whenever I enjoy the process of arranging flowers in a vase, the childhood image of my mum doing the same thing at our kitchen bench comes flooding back as if it were yesterday.

Each time I notice these family connections, I really let the moment land. I do this by taking a few deep breaths. I feel the sensations within my body and any emotions as they come and go. I remind myself that I am not alone. I am here doing this thing, on this day, because of the people who went before me. I allow this moment to anchor me into a deep sense of belonging and vitality.

Maybe over the years, you've been told you have your mother's eyes or your dad's long legs. Perhaps you get your creativity or your passion from your grandmother, your sense of humour or your sporting ability from your grandfather. Is the way you cook or express yourself rooted in your blood lines? Does your love of nature or animals come from a long family tradition?

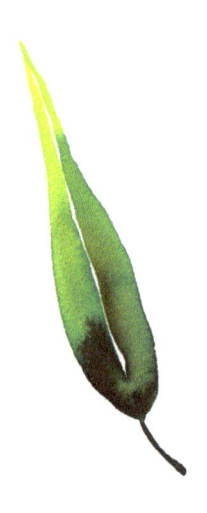

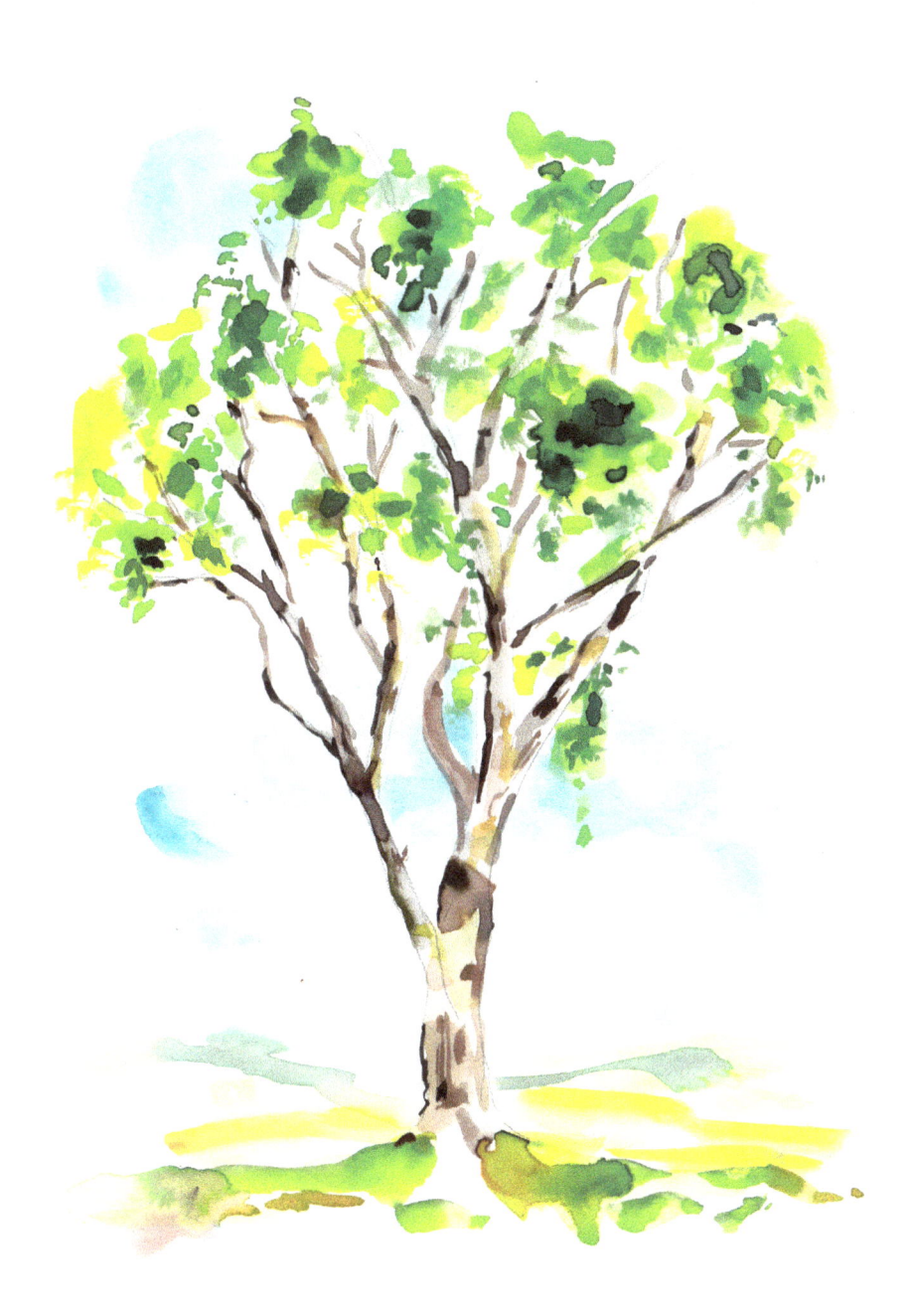

EXERCISE: AN ANTIDOTE TO FEELING ALONE

Over the next day, notice any activities, habits, or hobbies that remind you of a family member (past or present).

When you are engaging in this activity, really call to mind this person. Take a moment to imagine them doing this thing.

Notice any sensations in your body (perhaps of relaxation, softening, warmth, or energy).

Open to any emotions (maybe love, gratitude, joy, or even sadness).

Repeat silently in your mind:

Through my everyday actions I connect to my family past and present. I remember that I am not alone.

Sense into your ancestry. Acknowledge their lives, the moments of love and of sadness. Feel into their collective resilience.

Take a few deep breaths. Really encourage this moment of connection to land.

Look into the palms of your hands, allow the lines and the details to connect you to your ancestors.

Rub your hands together. Really feel the warmth and energy that is building within your hands.

Place your hands somewhere on your body that feels good for you (perhaps your cheeks, shoulders, or chest).

As you feel your own warmth, allow it to connect you to your family, your ancestors, and your own vitality.

Joy, demystified

Another way to feel more vital and alive is to intentionally cultivate more joy in your life. Joy can be defined and experienced in different ways. You might understand it as a positive emotion, an internal state, or as a wave of energy that washes over you, often taking you by surprise and filling you with gratitude, love, or wonder.

Our lives don't need to be perfect in order to experience joy. In fact, joy has a funny way of appearing when we least expect it. Like when you come home from work and your dog bounds up to see you, delight in their eyes. Or when you are driving, and you notice the first signs of spring.

When I'm teaching this ten pathways framework to people all around the world, I often ask students the question:

> Do you have enough joy in your life?
> The answer is usually a resounding 'no'.

After their no, a conversation about what gets in the way of more joy then follows. Often, the issue is — we're too busy! Most people are willing to acknowledge that when we move through our days consumed by our to-do lists, joy can fall under the radar. It's not that there aren't opportunities for joy, it's that our attention isn't there. I wonder if you can relate to this?

Over the years, both in my personal and professional life, I've discovered that when it comes to joy, there is something deeper at play than just our busyness. Can you guess? Much like gratitude, joy requires a sometimes uncomfortable combination of courage and vulnerability.

It's easy to assume that joy is a lighthearted, feel-good state. Joyful people are often depicted running through a field of yellow sunflowers or laughing with their friends or family without a care in the world. In truth, if we are to fully experience joy, we need to be brave enough to acknowledge the impermanent nature of our lives (I know you don't want to!).

As we discussed in the connection pathway earlier in this book, it can feel hard to accept that the people, circumstances, and things we love won't last forever. Really opening to joy involves sinking deep into the truth that our lives can be made more beautiful (not less) through their impermanent nature.

For example:

- Our children can feel more precious when we acknowledge that they won't always be this age or at this life stage.
- Our springtime garden can be more beautiful with the knowing that it won't last forever.
- Our morning run, walk, or yoga session can feel even more invigorating as we acknowledge that over time our bodies will age.
- A laugh with an old friend can feel even more sacred knowing that this friendship won't always be the same.

The problem is, we think we want to feel joyful ... but we're also a little scared of it. On some level, we know it's not a permanent emotion and that makes us feel vulnerable. For many of us, if a moment of joy naturally arises, we can't handle how strong it feels. In an instant — the love, gratitude, vitality, fear, and worry all swirl together creating an experience that feels too intense. So, we protect ourselves from all the feelings and from the wave of vulnerability.

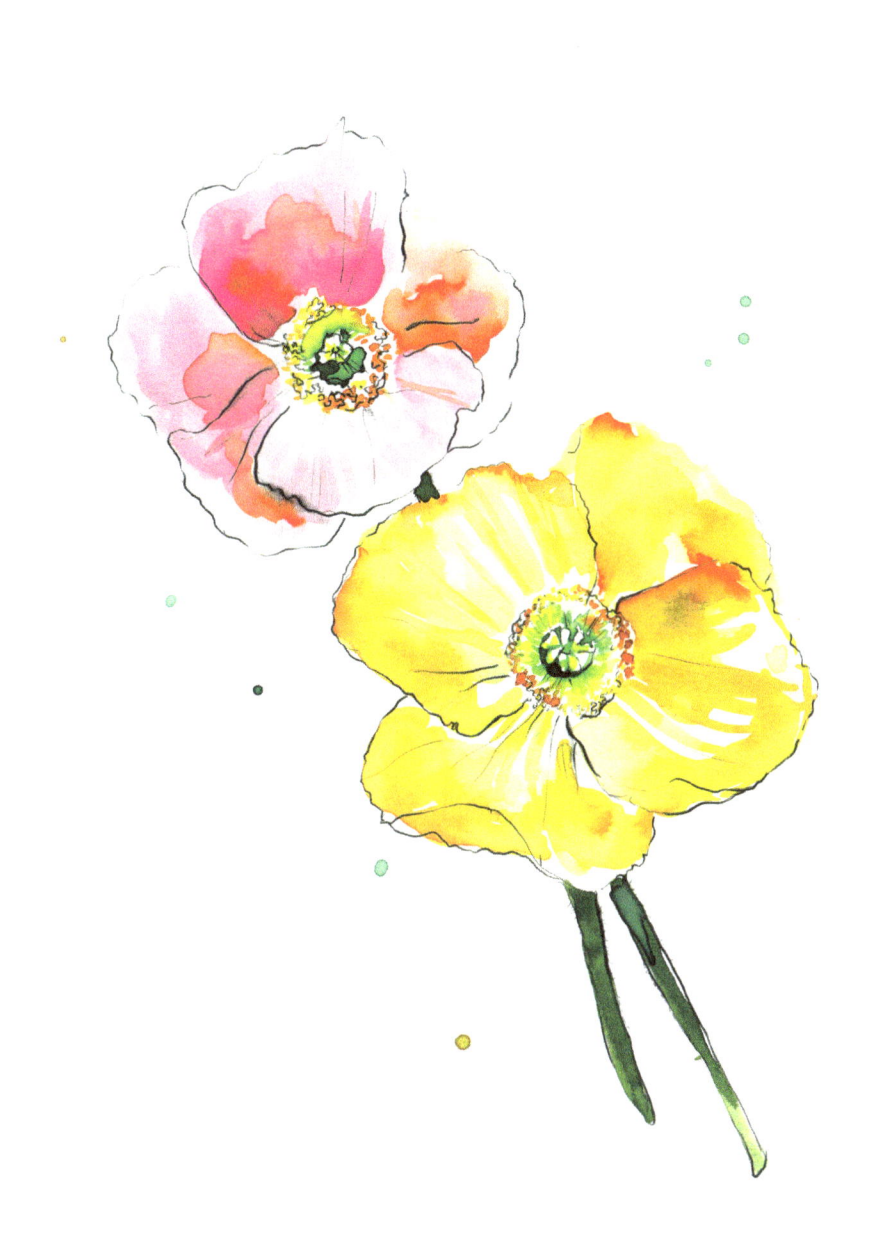

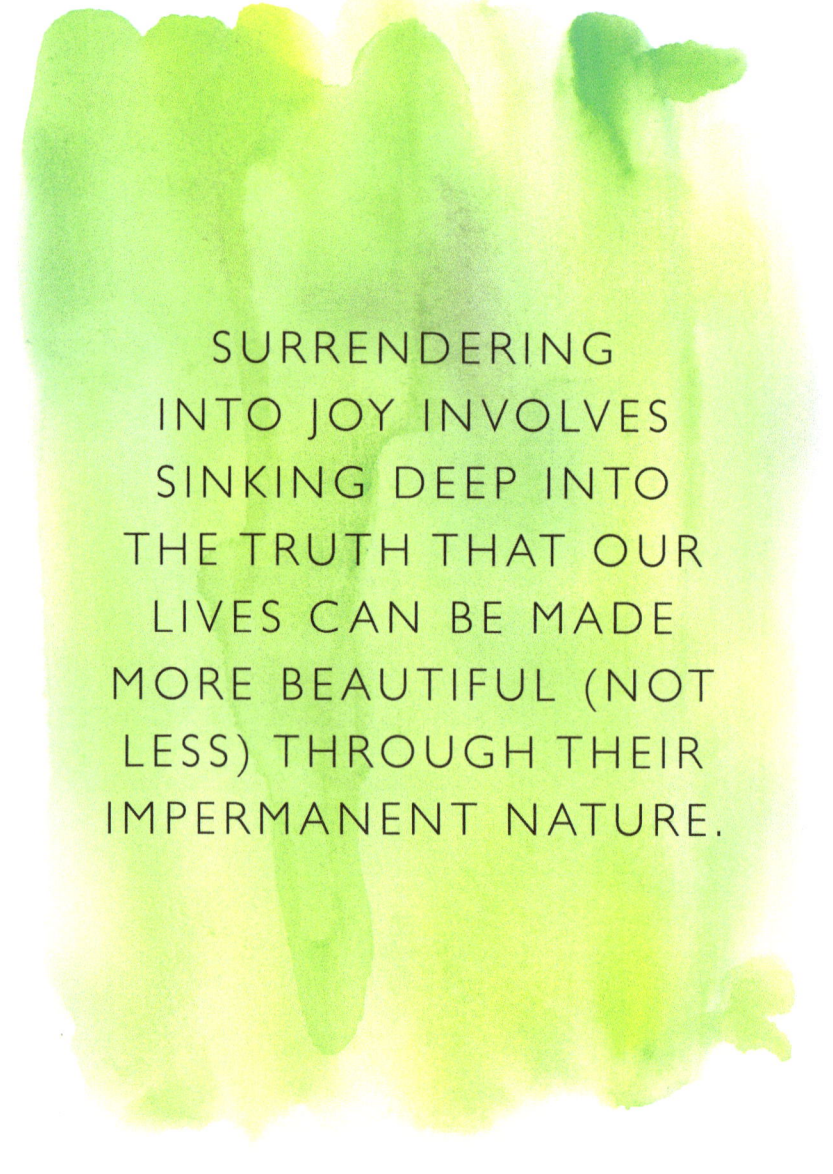

SURRENDERING INTO JOY INVOLVES SINKING DEEP INTO THE TRUTH THAT OUR LIVES CAN BE MADE MORE BEAUTIFUL (NOT LESS) THROUGH THEIR IMPERMANENT NATURE.

In her book, *Daring Greatly,* Dr Brené Brown talks about 'foreboding joy'. She explains this response to joy as a 'paradoxical dread that clamps down on momentary joyfulness'. Rather than sit with the cocktail of emotions that arise and the raw humanness of the experience, we focus instead on all the bad things that could happen. As she says, we 'dress-rehearse tragedy'.

Examples of foreboding joy include:

- When life is going well, when your children are happy and your parents are healthy, instead of surrendering into the love and sacredness of it all, your mind starts thinking: *This won't last forever, something bad is just around the corner, I'm sure.*
- When you receive praise at work or get a promotion, instead of celebrating the moment. you start visualising the day that you make a mistake or lose your strong footing. You dress-rehearse the moment you get caught out or people don't like you as much as they do now.
- When you are in a new relationship and the other person is really enjoying your company and accepting you for who you are, a little voice in the back of your mind is whispering: *This won't last, wait until they get to know the real you.*

Embracing a new version of happiness involves strengthening your capacity (and tolerance) for joy. Just as we have been learning to walk alongside our pain so that it may offer us gifts, so too must we learn to walk bravely alongside our joy. When you do, you'll feel more vital and alive.

The good news is, we can all get more comfortable with joy, including the vulnerability it often brings. Remember how, in the compassion pathway, we explored connecting with the wisdom and resilience found in our hearts? We can allow our hearts to hold us in the moments of joy too.

The first step is gratitude: get better at appreciating joyful moments. The second step is feeling safe in these moments. The easiest way to do this is to breathe. When you start to worry about the bad things that could happen next, take three deep breaths. Pause in the present moment and appreciate it in the now, rather than fearing for the future.

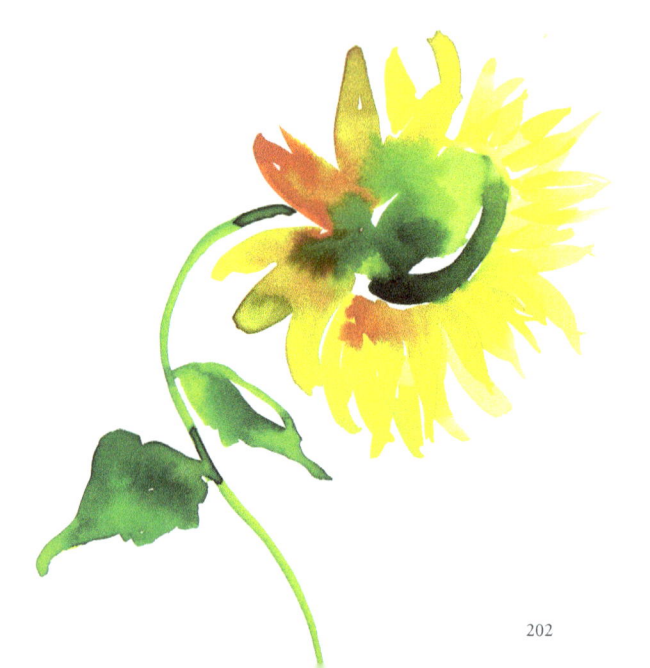

EXERCISE: AVOIDING THE JOY JITTERS

Close your eyes and take three deep breaths.

Cast your mind back to a time when you felt joy (perhaps recently or as a child).

Trust whatever memory emerges.

Take a minute to really bring the details to mind and heart.

Ask yourself these questions:

Who was there? What were you doing? Was it day or night? Were you inside or outside?

How did it feel in your body?

Stay with this memory and any sensations or emotions that present themselves for five breaths.

Notice how even though this specific moment in time is gone, you can still feel its gifts.

Reflect on how the moment was impermanent but the joy lives on in your memory and in your heart.

Offer gratitude to this moment and to those in it.

Notice also how you are safe to reflect on this moment and to enjoy it without getting hooked into the energy of foreboding joy, or worst-case scenarios.

Take a deep breath into your heart. Feel into its strength and sense of resilience.

Repeat silently in your mind:

I am safe to embrace the moments of joy in my life. I welcome joy.

Well done, you have just strengthened your capacity for joy.

PATHWAY NINE: CONFIDENCE

Finding your place on the stage called life

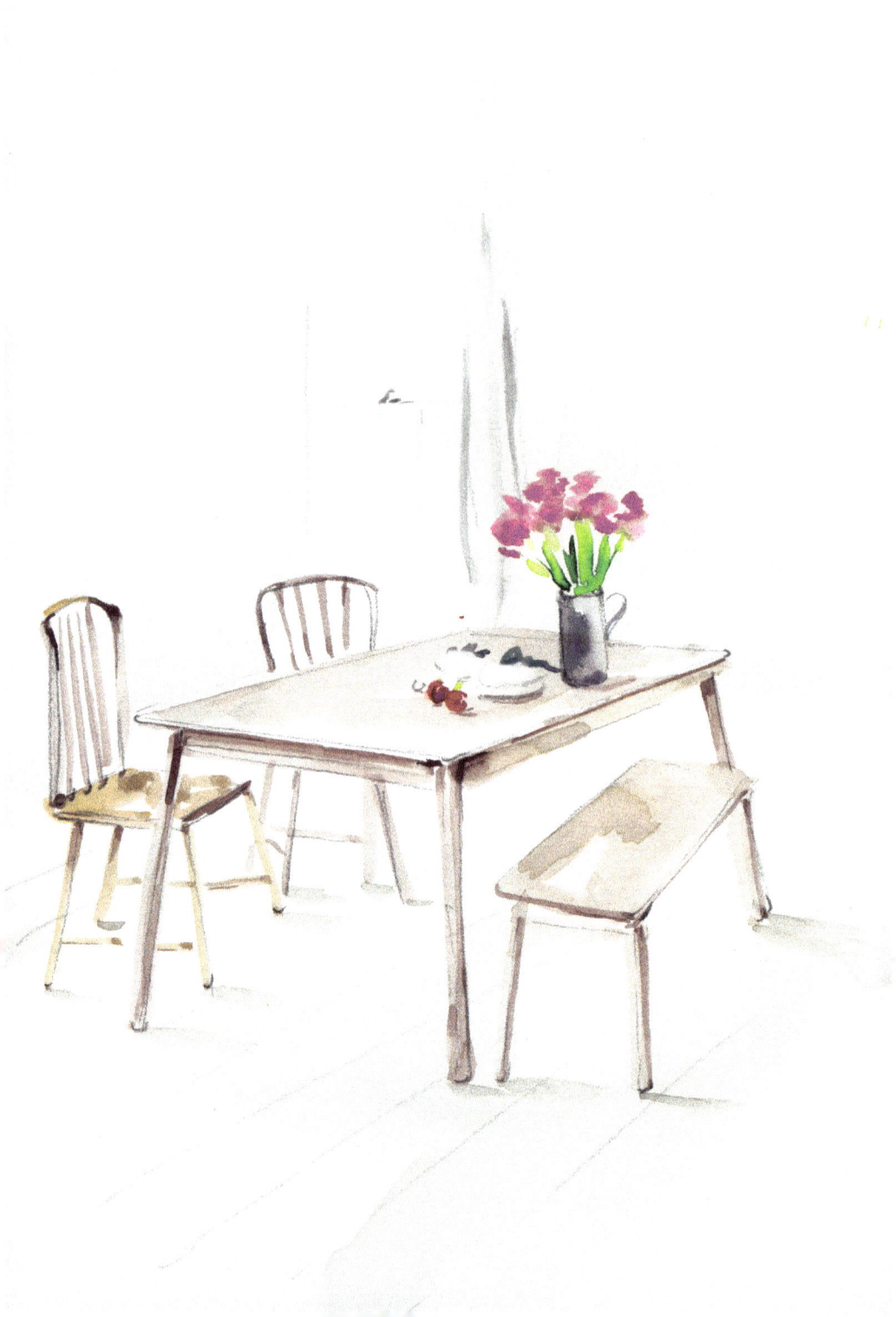

Our challenges are rich opportunities to become more, not less, confident.

It surprises me how often, as an adult, I find myself thinking about our family dinner table growing up. I can still picture clearly the tapered legs that were a magnet for our little bare feet (if I had a dollar for every time I stubbed my toe!). I remember the splashes of paint, the small holes, and old pieces of sticky tape forever adhered to the sides of the table; a reminder of birthday presents wrapped lovingly years before.

Every night, Mum would ask one of us three children to tidy and set the table. This job would include rearranging all the random pieces of paper, books, and bits and pieces into a consolidated pile down one end of the table. We all knew when my brother had undertaken this family chore, because the pile was always on a precarious angle, and the knives and forks were on the wrong sides. He blamed it on being a left-hander, but I'm a 'lefty' too and somehow managed to do it right.

I remember the family dynamics, as reliable as those solid table legs. Every night at dinner my older sister would capture the family's attention by sharing stories from her day. She had a natural ability for accents and irony. My brother found his unique place as the only boy, safely nestled between two girls. Most nights I sat in silence. I listened. I observed. I'm not sure exactly when my quietness, my gentle ability to pay attention to my surroundings earned me the label of shy.

AMAZINGLY, IT'S
THE CHALLENGES
WE FACE – BE IT
PHYSICAL, MENTAL,
OR EMOTIONAL –
THAT CAN BE A HELP,
NOT A HINDRANCE,
TO OUR CONFIDENCE.

As with so many childhood traits, the lines between label and identity became blurred like chalk drawings on the pavement. Over the years, I settled without question into the belief that I was shy. I wrapped myself up in this identity like a warm and familiar blanket. I allowed it to protect me throughout my teenage years and well into my twenties.

I'm sure being the youngest also played a part in my 'shyness'. Today, I see it play out in my own family — my youngest son, desperately trying to talk, but often being drowned out by his older brothers. In these moments, I smile as I remember one of my mother's favourite expressions, 'Never underestimate the impact of sibling position, darl!' This was her response every time I complained about my brother or sister.

After those family dinners where I sat in silence, I would hide away in my bedroom writing poetry and song lyrics. Growing up in the 1980s, I loved recording these poems and songs onto my pink cassette player.

I can still remember how heavy the red record button felt underneath my small finger. In these moments, I was held by delight and fear in equal measure. A rush of pleasure washed over me as I tapped into an internal spring of self-expression and creativity. This was met by a rumbling anxiety that my older brother may find these tapes and hold them for ransom. It's not totally surprising, I now record meditations for a living.

We all carry the experiences, family dynamics, and in some cases, trauma from our childhood into our adult lives. There's no escaping it. When we are young, we develop protective habits in order to feel safe, loved, and accepted. Over time, this conditioning morphs into our identity as adults. Our desire to please, to make others happy, to be competent or capable, caring or kind all have origins within our childhood. Our procrastination, our perfectionism, our fear of being alone, judged, or not enough also have roots deep in our past.

As world-renowned neuroscientist, Dr Rick Hanson, writes in his book *Resilient*, 'Thousands of little episodes in which a child's self-expression and assertiveness are accepted and managed skilfully — or not — add up over time to shape a person one way or another.' If we want to be happy as adults, we must be willing to reflect on our childhood with both curiosity and compassion.

Fast-forward thirty-five years and here I am, forty-something years old, still gently observing and writing from the heart, still giving voice to my inner world and sharing my reflections on life into a microphone on my own.

I've moved from my two-tone pink bedroom into a professional recording studio. I've also moved from feeling fearful of being heard, to deeply okay with being visible in this way, knowing that people in over forty countries are listening to my words.

Ironically, I owe much of my new-found confidence to my chronic illness and the fact that I had to become my own advocate. All those times I asked for another test, a second opinion, or an alternative treatment plan acted like building blocks on my tower of inner strength. The moments I chose to trust my own body more than the physiotherapist, and my gut instinct more than the specialist. The times when the pain was all consuming but I reminded myself that just like the sun, I would rise again to face another day. All these moments, whilst hard, edged me closer to a version of confidence that was filled with courage and self-trust.

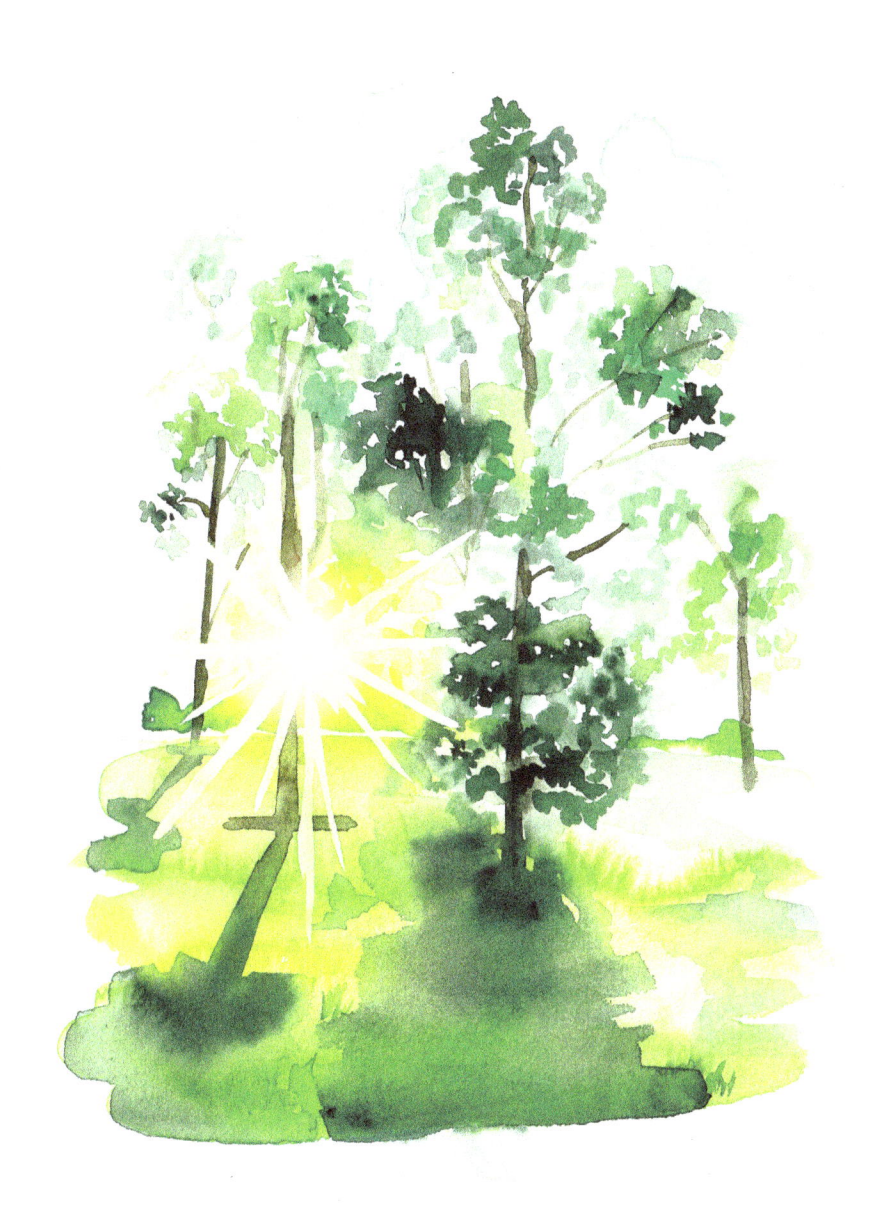

Amazingly, it's the challenges we face, be it physical, mental, or emotional, that can be a help, not a hindrance, to our confidence. When you have to advocate for yourself, whether it's in relation to getting a diagnosis or treatment plan, ending a romantic or platonic relationship, or standing up for yourself at work, confidence naturally grows.

In order to grow, we need to let go

Growing up, I would tell myself I needed to be more like the girls who put their hand up for the lead in the school play or sang the solo in the school choir. Given my fear of being the centre of attention, this story I told myself made me anxious and full of dread. This inner belief, that in order to feel confident, I had to do things that frightened me and didn't feel natural, sat heavy on my young self.

As I grew up, I continued to tell myself that I needed to be more, to add to myself in order to feel confident. Sometimes these stories defied all logic and probability. Like the one about how I'd feel confident when my legs were longer!

I now know that these subconscious beliefs are very common. I hear it all the time in my work. People from all different ages, life stages, and backgrounds are plagued with this internal dialogue. You might smile as you see yourself in these stories:

- The mother who tells herself she'll feel more confident when her family listens to her more or when the kids are older and she finally has time to explore her own interests and dreams.
- The young person who is sure that confidence will come knocking when they get their first job, gain that qualification or make new friends.

- The loyal staff member who is waiting for that promotion, praise or recognition before they feel appreciated and self-assured.
- The person who moves through their day believing that getting fit, losing a few pounds and finding a new partner will help them feel more comfortable in their own skin.
- The older person who is sure they've made too many mistakes in the past to ever believe in themselves, or that the confidence ship has sailed for them.

It's so easy to get in the habit of telling ourselves that confidence will arrive like an express-post parcel at the front door when we add more to who we are. Whilst there's nothing wrong with wanting to improve and add to your skill set and experience, the problem with these 'I'll be confident when …' stories is that they're based on a belief that right here, right now, you are not enough.

When our actions come from a foundation of lack, of not 'enoughness', they never offer us the satisfaction we desire. It's like we're pouring sand into a bucket with a hole in the bottom. It never fills up no matter what we do.

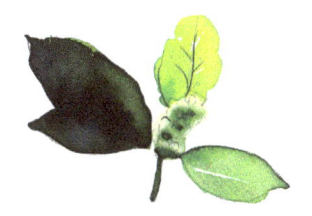

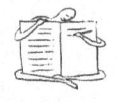

EXERCISE: WHAT'S YOUR STORY?

The first step in reimagining confidence is shining the light of awareness onto your 'I'll be confident when ...' stories. As we've discussed many times throughout this book — with awareness, we create space. From here you'll be able to see these stories with greater perspective, and ultimately, let them go.

Grab a pen and paper.

Write on the top of the page 'I'll be confident when ...'

Make a list of all the stories you tell yourself.

When you get to the end of the list, take a deep breath, and go deeper. Write down the stories that feel ridiculous, unrealistic, or irrational.

Read over the list with a sense of curiosity, non-judgement, and maybe even humour.

As you see the words on the paper, allow yourself to feel separate from these stories.

Really sink into the idea that these words do not define you.

You may like to rip this piece of paper into tiny pieces or even burn it (safely!).

Notice any sense of relief and freedom that this activity brings.

Repeat this writing exercise whenever you feel old stories owning you.

Realise your confidence is here for you ... today!

'Enoughness' as an adult

As we've discussed throughout this book, taking time to reflect on your childhood, and the beliefs and identities you formed about yourself, can be both illuminating and healing. The memories that surface don't need to be dramatic or painful. Often, it's the small and seemingly random moments that etch their way into our being and shape who we are and how we see the world.

Like the time your aunty told you that you were too loud or your mother told you to not get so emotional. Maybe it's the moment your sports teacher said you weren't good enough to make the team. Or that time, during puberty, when you felt too tall or short, too chubby or skinny.

Perhaps when you were young you compared yourself to your siblings, cousins, or friends — these comparisons making you feel insecure. Maybe these comparisons didn't come from you, but your mother or father ('Why can't you be more like your brother or sister?').

When we are brave enough to sit with these memories, they can offer great insight and help us understand our adult selves more fully. It won't happen overnight, but with time, understanding, and patience, you can loosen the grip these childhood memories have over you. As you do this, you'll notice yourself feeling more confident.

EXERCISE: CONNECTING THE DOTS

Find somewhere comfortable to sit and close your eyes.

Take a few deep breaths.

Feel the places within your body that rest on the surface beneath you. Soften into this sense of physical support.

Gently direct your mind back to your childhood. You might like to picture your family home growing up or the things you liked to do.

Without trying too hard, allow a memory to surface. Notice the details. Who was there? What were you doing? How did you feel?

Offer this younger version of you whatever they need in the moment, perhaps a smile, some reassurance that they are loveable or enough as they are. Maybe they just need your warm-hearted attention.

Stay with this moment of connection for a few breaths. Notice any sensations in your body, perhaps a sense of softening, relief, or warmth.

Allow this memory and moment of connection to help you understand your adult self a little more.

Open into any clues or insights. Trust in this moment.

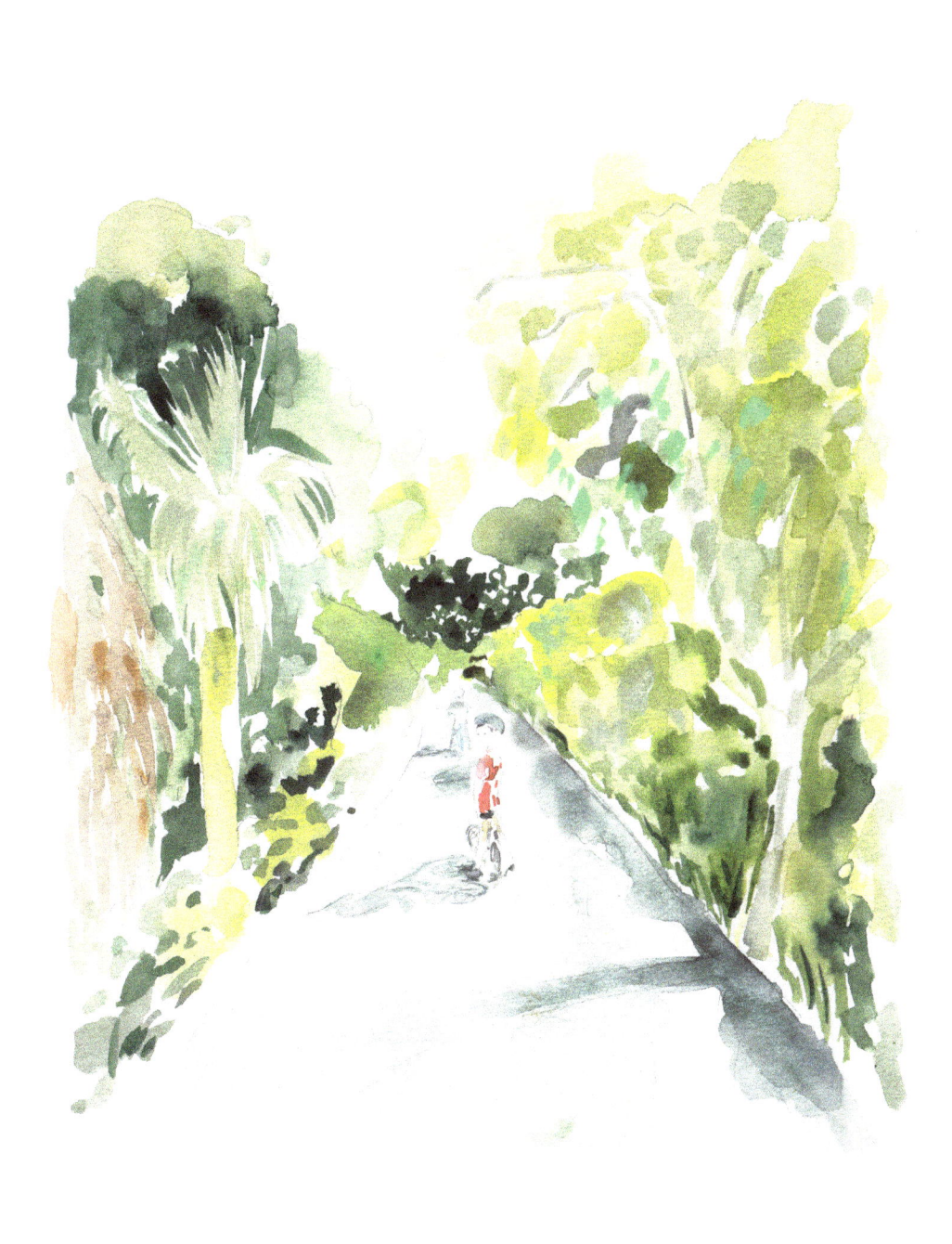

From comparison to compassion

We all know people who, in our minds, we perceive as naturally confident. We notice these people light up a room, capturing people's attention with engaging stories about their lives or by sharing their plans for the future.

Professionally, we see them speaking up in meetings and promoting themselves on social media. As an outsider, it seems as if these people are always trying new things and grabbing opportunities without hesitation or doubt. We imagine that their family life is fulfilling and rewarding; that they are never weighed down by the fear of not being good enough or being judged.

This is where the comparisons creep in. We begin to judge ourselves for not chasing our dreams, speaking up, asking for what we need, or having clear boundaries. We wonder why our family isn't as close as theirs, why our work isn't as rewarding.

These comparisons never lead to us feeling confident. For the most part, they add another log to the fire of insecurity that's slowly burning within us. On the off-chance that our comparisons make us feel 'better' than another person, this inauthentic rush of confidence is fleeting. It's quickly replaced by a feeling of unease as we fear this person may catch up to us, or even worse, overtake us in this unhealthy game of comparison. It's hard to relax on a wobbly pedestal!

So how do you break free from the unhealthy habit of comparison? By offering compassion — to yourself and the other person.

At first it might feel hard, forced, or even insincere, but trust that over time it will feel easier and more authentic. You might even notice your body relax, your perspective broaden, and your self-esteem grow. From here, you'll really begin to believe that there is enough love, success, joy, and happiness for us all.

Try taking a deep breath and repeating one of these phrases silently in your mind the next time you notice yourself pulled into the comparison trap:

- I know you are human just like me.
- I wish you well.
- There is enough love/success/happiness/recognition for both of us.
- I trust that I am where I am meant to be.

EXERCISE: LOVE THY COMPETITION

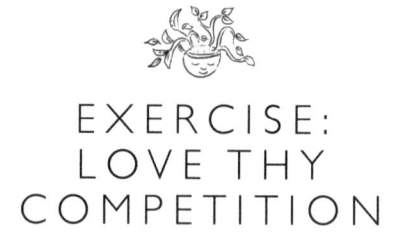

Begin gently by calling to mind someone you have been comparing yourself to recently.

For a few breaths, open to the possibility that this person is human just like you.

Really allow the idea that they too have moments of self-doubt, fears of not being worthy, or concerns for their future to settle over your awareness.

Allow this possibility to relax your body, calm your mind, and soften your heart.

You may even like to wish this person well. Repeat silently in your mind:

I wish you well.

Take a deep breath into the liberating idea that there is enough love, success, joy, and happiness for us all.

Smile, knowing that this small yet radical act of moving from comparison to compassion will ripple into your relationships and your life.

Keep this exercise in your toolkit — always there for you.

Just as there is enough happiness for everyone, there is enough pain too! What I mean is that no-one is free from discomfort, whether chronic or short-term. After I received my diagnosis, I would look at people exercising in the park or jogging by the beach with both amazement and envy. Thoughts like: *How can this person move their body like that and not experience pain? I wish I was pain free like they are*, swirling around in my mind. With the passage of time, I can see how these comparisons only made me feel more alone — eroding my confidence even more.

After about one month of consistently offering myself and others my compassion (using the phrases and exercise previously mentioned), I noticed a shift within me. I began to see these people (the ones doing all the things I couldn't) as human just like me. I could really 'feel' into the possibility that they also had challenges to face. This realisation, that we are all walking around with hidden scars and burdens that others cannot see, was strangely comforting. It allowed me to feel more connected to family, friends, and strangers. Once again, my pain offered me an unexpected gift — the opportunity to step more fully into the shared experience of being human.

I hope as you're reading this book, you're beginning to see how your challenges, far from being obstacles to confidence, can be powerful opportunities to advocate for yourself, cultivate self-belief, and move beyond the stories that no longer serve you towards a greater sense of shared connection.

On the days when the old narratives creep back in and the inner doubt casts a shadow over your awareness, remember that these feelings are impermanent. Remind yourself that they too will pass and that you don't need to cling onto them or let them define or overwhelm you.

PATHWAY TEN: ACCEPTANCE

Pain x resistance = suffering

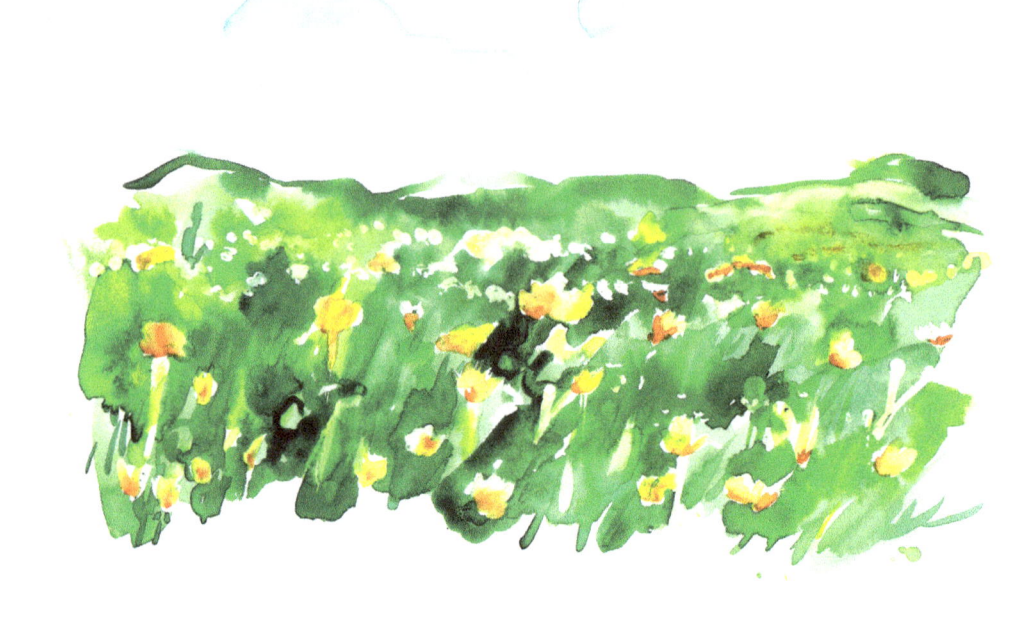

Small moments of acceptance are enough to alter your inner and outer landscape.

If you're like the thousands of people around the world who have explored this ten pathways framework with me, the word acceptance probably brings up all sorts of inner dialogue.

- If I accept my circumstances, how will I improve my life?
- If I accept my relationships, will people walk all over me or take me for granted?
- If I accept myself, what will motivate me to better myself and work towards everything I want and desire?

These questions highlight a commonly held fear in people of all ages and life stages; that acceptance (of yourself or your life) will lead to 'resignation'. So many of us hold the belief (either consciously or subconsciously) that if we accept ourselves or our lives then we will stop trying. We will settle for an average existence: unsatisfying work, unrewarding relationships, and a life that feels ordinary.

Take a moment to imagine such a person, full of resignation (and even self-pity). Perhaps their shoulders are hunched over, and their eyes are fixated on the ground. Maybe they appear withdrawn, closed off to the world, or willing to let life happen to them. They carry with them the energy of defeat, even hopelessness. With these visuals in mind, it's no wonder people aren't lining up for a ticket to the acceptance pathway.

Here's a hard-won truth I'd like to share with you after years of living with (and resisting) chronic physical and emotional pain. True acceptance is the opposite of resignation, it's actually empowering and energising. You may be wondering how it can feel so light and liberating. The answer is simple: acceptance involves letting go of the heavy weight that is resistance.

The weight of resistance

When we resist ourselves and our lives it's like wearing a 20kg backpack all day, every day. Except, in this case, this metaphorical backpack is filled with our *thoughts*. You know the ones:

> I can't believe they said/did that.
> I wish that didn't happen.
> It's so unfair.
> Why me?
> I need to be more kind/thoughtful/patient.
> I'm not successful/interesting/beautiful/fit enough.
> I need more love/money/recognition in my life.

Our resistance backpacks are filled with heavy *emotions* too:

> Remorse.
> Shame.
> Guilt.
> Anger.
> Jealously.
> Envy.

They can also hold *energies*:

> Regretting.
> Ruminating.
> Wanting.
> Striving.
> Yearning.

Carrying around these heavy thoughts, emotions, and energies impacts our bodies, minds, and hearts. It can also affect our personal identities and the way we interact with others and our lives. With people I've taken through the ten pathways framework, I've seen resistance show up in different ways. It can:

- Cause physical stress in our bodies including tension, tightness, and pain.
- Alter our posture so that our chest (and heart) become closed off and we can't access states like compassion, gratitude, kindness, or forgiveness.
- Promote repetitive thinking that narrows our perspective and ability to creatively problem-solve and seek out new opportunities.
- Encourage us to avoid our emotions.
- Lead to long-term feelings of self-doubt, insecurity, and low self-worth.
- Encourage habits like perfectionism, people-pleasing, and procrastination.
- Result in us trying to control and micromanage the small details of our lives and our relationships.
- Reduce our capacity to find meaning in, and learn from, our pain, challenges, and setbacks.

Becoming familiar with your own unique habits of resistance (the way you frequently regret the past, worry about the future, or tell yourself that you need to be more) is the first step on the pathway of acceptance. You can begin this line of enquiry by asking yourself these three questions:

1. What thoughts, emotions or energies am I carrying right now?

2. Where in my body do I feel their weight?

3. What happens to my perspective or outlook when I carry these burdens?

The second step is to see acceptance as a fluid and dynamic experience rather than a permanent or concrete state.

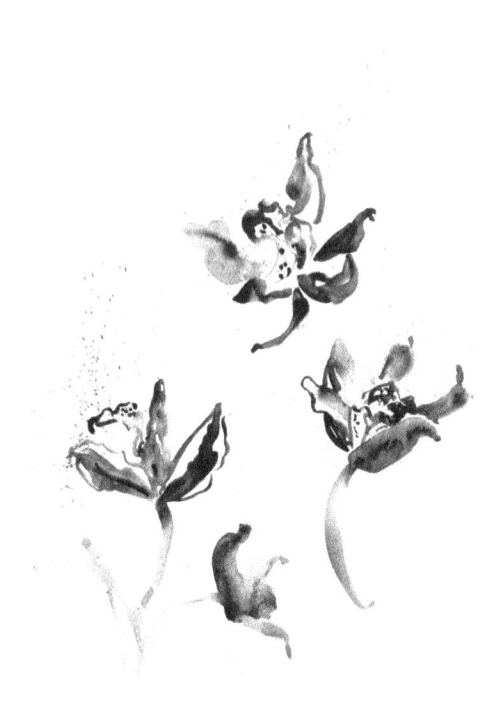

EXERCISE: A BREAK FROM YOUR BACKPACK

Imagine now that you are wearing a backpack. Notice how heavy it feels on your body. Notice also how it makes your shoulders slouch and your chest close off. With this heavy weight, your eyes become fixated on the ground, and you cannot see the wider environment.

Take a deep breath. Open to the possibility that this is what resistance does. It creates tension in your physical and emotional body and narrows your perspective.

Now imagine that you are taking off the heavy backpack. Notice (or imagine) your body feeling lighter and more open. Pay attention to how, without the heavy backpack, your posture straightens, and your chest opens. It's possible to look up and notice your surroundings.

This is the energy of acceptance.

Take a deep breath into any lightness or freedom that is here for you.

Repeat silently in your mind:

It feels good to let go of the weight that is resistance.

I'm safe to accept myself and my life, one moment at a time.

Acceptance comes in waves

Unless you are a Buddhist monk living in a monastery, chances are, acceptance isn't a state you'll be able to cultivate on a permanent basis (and that's okay!). As we move into the final pathway and chapter of this book, I hope you're already beginning to feel a shift in your life. However, I also know that, despite amazing progress, this is when our inner critic and perfectionist can start to creep in as we ask ourselves: *But why do I still have moments where I feel resistant? Why am I not walking around in a constant state of Zenfulness?*

In our fast-paced, productivity-driven world, it's natural to have moments of resistance as you move through your days. Feeling overwhelmed by your inbox, frustrated by a delayed train, or disappointed that your kids didn't eat their dinner are all natural responses to everyday life.

Redefining happiness isn't about accepting everything all the time. Nor will it protect you from ever experiencing hurt, disappointment, or regret. I hope that ten chapters into this book, you've realised that true happiness isn't about living in a constant, idealistic nirvana.

It is more about learning to pause every now and then and to *notice* what you are resisting. As we've discussed many times throughout this book, awareness creates space, and ultimately, freedom. Through this radical act of noticing, we are more able to let the resistance go (even if only for a short moment) and invite acceptance to fill its place.

When we acknowledge that the energies of resistance and acceptance flow in waves (and that we have the power to invite them in or let them go), we are more able to understand and forgive ourselves when life feels wobbly.

Sometimes, despite our best intentions, it feels like we are taking one step forward and two steps back. For example:

- The newly separated person who enjoys a few weeks feeling positive about their future and then wakes one day furious with their ex-partner and wishes they had never met.
- The middle-aged person who, in good grace, takes on the role of caring for their elderly parents, but every now and then feels frustrated and resentful.
- The new parents who love and enjoy their young children but sometimes fantasise about undisturbed sleep, freedom, and life before kids.
- The younger person who experiences greater confidence after getting fit, eating well, and meditating regularly and then suddenly has a period of anxiety and low self-esteem.

Personal growth (and life) is not linear — twists and turns are a natural part of being human. When we strengthen our capacity to create moments of acceptance within the messiness, to feel our scars with a warm-hearted presence, life feels easier and more enjoyable.

EXERCISE: LIGHTEN YOUR LOAD

Grab a pen and paper. Find a comfortable place to sit. Take three deep breaths. Think of something in your life that you are resisting. Choose something small or medium, like a conversation where you said something you now regret or a disappointment that you've been holding on to. Follow this six-step process to lighten your load.

1. Describe this situation in a few sentences. *Right now, I know that I am resisting...*

2. Write down all the thoughts you are having about this situation that feel like resistance (they might begin with phrases like: *I wish I didn't...* or, *I can't believe...*).

3. Write down the emotions that surface when you are caught in these thoughts and the energy of resistance (for example: guilt, shame, resentment, embarrassment, regret, resentment, anger, rage).

4. Cast your eye over what you have written. Notice the weight of these thoughts and emotions.

5. Remember the exercise we did earlier in this chapter when we imagined taking off our metaphorical backpacks? Visualise it now.

6. Now take some time to write about this situation from a more accepting position. What thoughts would you have? What emotions would you experience? How would you feel about yourself and your life?

Well done, you just cultivated a moment of acceptance!

You can't teach self-acceptance

As we take the final steps on our tenth pathway towards a more real and sustainable version of happiness, we are offered the greatest challenge of all: learning to accept ourselves just as we are.

As a meditation teacher who specialises in helping people cultivate more open and friendly relations with themselves, I know that it's not possible to 'teach' someone to accept themselves. But people certainly try! Social media is filled with quotes like 'you deserve your own love' and 'embrace your imperfections'.

I imagine that most of these statements are met with scepticism, as no-one likes to be told to accept themselves. The practice of feeling comfortable in one's own skin must originate from within (a cliché but so accurate).

So, I'll save you the pep talk that you are perfectly imperfect. I won't try to convince you that self-acceptance acts like a magic wand, dissolving all your insecurities, inner judgements, and fear. Instead, I'll remind you of four practices you've already explored throughout this book that may help you move closer towards your own unique expression of self-acceptance.

Awareness

You can pause anywhere, anytime and notice your thoughts. Are you replaying or regretting something you said or did? Are you worrying that you aren't good enough or that you need to be more? You can circuit-break these thoughts by engaging your senses and reminding yourself that you are safe. From here, you can ask these thoughts: *Are you kind, do you help me be the person I long to be?*

Compassion

Pay attention to the way you speak to yourself. Remember that harsh words create stress in our bodies and close off our hearts. Learn to identify the habits and patterns of your inner critic. Commit to responding to this inner aspect with a voice that feels more supportive, your inner ally.

Perspective

When you feel like you aren't enough and people won't accept you, when you notice yourself getting caught in habits of people-pleasing and perfectionism, pause and breathe deeply. Notice if you are being overly hard on yourself, and as best you can, offer yourself understanding and forgiveness. Identify those self-imposed high expectations and if possible, soften them. Become aware of when you are taking things personally and open to seeing things from a broader and more balanced perspective.

Connection

When you are being hard on yourself or feeling insecure, spend time outside. Notice the perfect timing of nature: the ebb and flow, the creation and destruction. Open to the truth that life is always changing and that nothing lasts forever. Allow this recognition of impermanence to remind you that you won't always feel this way.

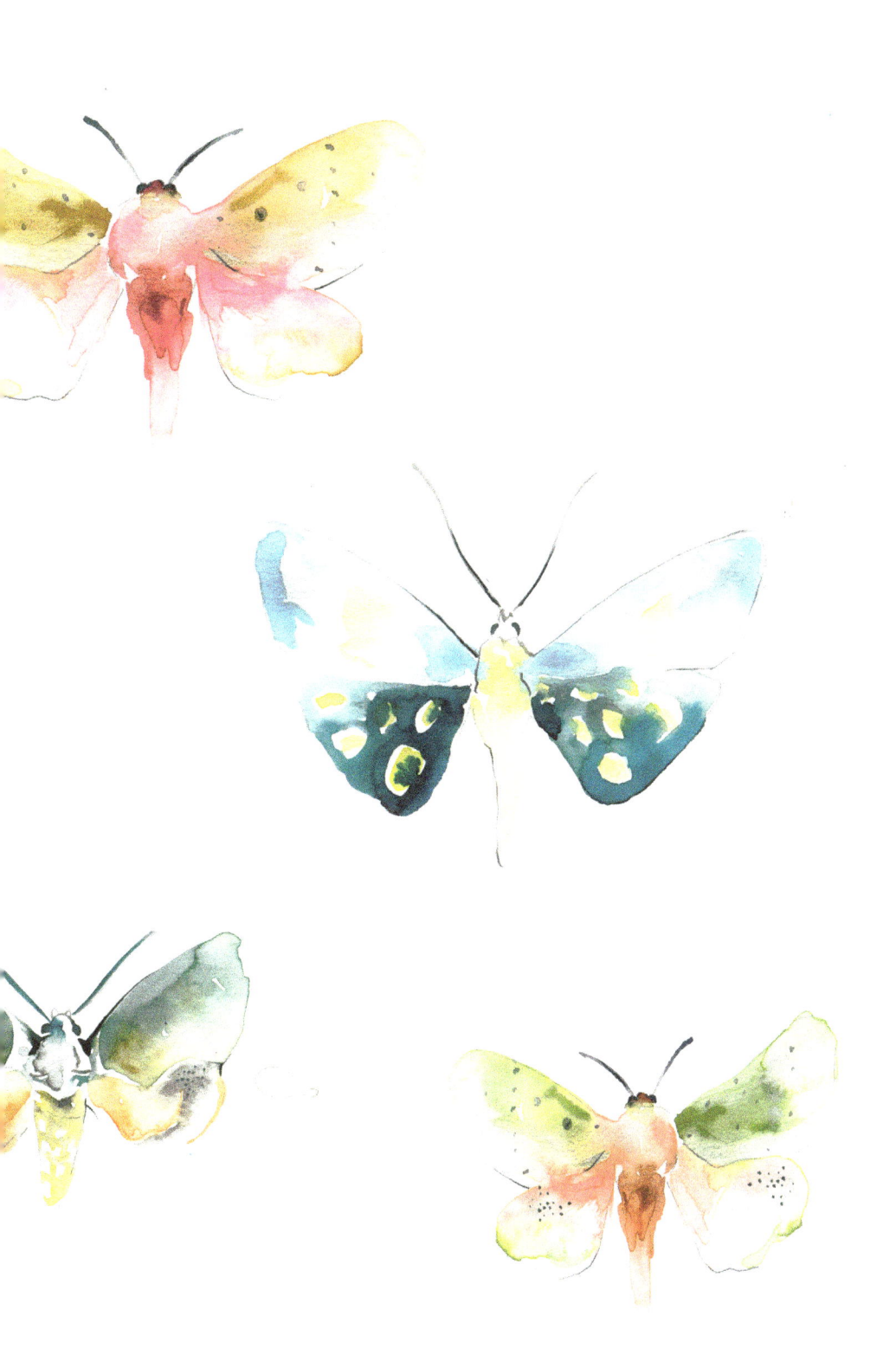

You already know how to pause and notice the ways you are resisting yourself. You have practiced how to offer yourself supporting phrases when your inner critic becomes loud. You know how to ask yourself different questions that will create a more friendly dynamic within you.

Remember also that self-acceptance doesn't need to be a permanent state and it's enough to cultivate small moments of inner friendliness. Over time, these moments will bring you into the landscape of your heart, the place where you can dare to imagine: *What would my life look and feel like if I accepted myself exactly as I am?*

My pain, my companion

As I write this, I've lived with chronic pain for seven years. I've raised my children through chronic pain. I've built a successful meditation app through chronic pain. I've written this book through chronic pain. I've also helped thousands of other people deal with their chronic pain, both emotional and physical. People often ask me:

> When did you decide to accept your chronic pain diagnosis (and the possibility that physical pain may be a permanent feature of your life)?

> The short answer is: I didn't decide. It just happened slowly over time.

During the first few months after my formal fibromyalgia diagnosis, all I could think of was the doctor's words: 'There is no pill you can take for this condition. There is also no cure. All you can do is change the way you respond to the pain.' During this time, I practiced all the strategies we've discussed in this chapter to find even a tiny drop of acceptance. I knew deep in my heart that resisting my diagnosis was hurting me more than the physical pain itself.

Over those lonely months, I became an expert at noticing when I was resisting my pain and when my metaphorical backpack felt the heaviest. I became curious about the type of thoughts and emotions I experienced when I was caught in the energy of resistance. Thoughts like, *It's not fair,* and, *I don't know how much more I can handle.* Emotions like anger, disappointment, and loneliness.

I observed how resistance felt in my body and what it did to my outlook on life. I offered the physical tension and the growing fear my attention. I offered myself kindness and compassion. I stayed present to my entire experience without judgement. I didn't push anything away.

From here, I was able to cultivate small moments of acceptance both for the way I was feeling in that moment and for the bigger picture of my chronic pain condition. I trusted in the healing power of these tiny islands of safety and ease. Over time, I could feel a dual sense of softening and opening within me. The pain was still there but I was no longer at war with it.

When I noticed the inner shift from resistance to acceptance, I encouraged the moment to land (remember we talked about this in the gratitude pathway?) by closing my eyes and imagining the horizon line. I pictured the exact point where the land meets the sky. I imaged this horizon line travelling as far as my eye could see in both directions. I took a deep breath into this sense of expansiveness. I allowed it to soften my body, warm my heart and broaden my perspective. From here, it felt possible to understand my pain in a totally new way.

I realised, without a doubt, that I get to choose what meaning I assign to my pain. From that moment on, I chose to understand my pain in this empowering way:

- Physical pain is my body's way of communicating with me.
- When I experience pain it's my body telling me that I have lost my way, that I have strayed from what really matters.
- Fibromyalgia is my body's way of guiding me home.

So now, each time I experience a pain episode, I take a few deep breaths and ask my pain: *What are you here to teach me? What would you have me know?*

Over the years my pain has had a lot to say. Here are some of my favourite pieces of wisdom:

- It's okay to be vulnerable.
- You are tired, stop pushing yourself so hard.
- Take an afternoon nap!
- Listen to your heart, it told you to stop eating meat!
- Stop worrying about what other people think of you.
- You are safe to make mistakes.

It's amazing to think that these small moments of acceptance were enough to totally transform my relationship with my chronic pain (and my world view). May this be a reminder to you that whatever pain is here for you, however trapped, disempowered, or afraid you feel, the small moments do add up. I hope you'll have the courage and the commitment to weave small islands of acceptance into your daily life.

My experience of allowing pain to alter my world view and pave the way for greater happiness is not unique. In my work I often hear from people who are allowing their challenges to open their eyes to a totally new way of living. Grief, job loss, separation, sickness, and even anxiety have put under the microscope what really matters and encouraged people to live differently.

In psychology, the idea that people who endure adversity can often experience positive growth afterwards is called post-traumatic growth. This theory was developed by psychologists Dr Richard Tedeschi and Dr Lawrence Calhoun in the mid-1990s. Their research highlights that after adversity, people can develop new understandings of themselves, the world they live in, and how they want to live and relate to other people.

Sarah Wilson, in her book, *First, We Make The Beast Beautiful,* describes this possibility powerfully when stating, 'The more we are shaken, the more our former selves and assumptions are blown apart, the fresher the growth.'

Your challenges don't need to be extraordinary in order to produce a shift within you. You can use your everyday stumbling blocks as opportunities to expand your world view. So how can you experience this shift? You can begin as I did, by befriending the horizon line.

EXERCISE: THE HORIZON LINE

Gaze at the illustration of the horizon line. Enjoy a few deep breaths as you take in the small details. Notice how it makes you feel.

Close your eyes and continue to imagine a horizon line (either this one or one of your own).

Trust that as you focus on this horizon line, your body will naturally relax, and your perspective will expand.

Soften the space above your eyes. Allow your shoulders to drop. Relax your belly.

Bring to mind a challenge you are facing at the moment (something you would like to feel more accepting of).

Offer this situation or circumstance a few deep breaths, almost as if you are breathing the horizon line deep into your body.

Breathe in acceptance.

Breathe out acceptance.

Ask this challenge:

What are you here to teach me? What would you have me know?

Listen. Trust.

Remember, you get to choose what meaning you assign to your challenges and your pain.

May you have the courage to find a meaning that moves you closer to inner happiness.

(Gratitude to Phillip Loft for teaching me how to connect to the horizon.)

THE MORE WE ARE
SHAKEN, THE MORE
OUR FORMER SELVES
AND ASSUMPTIONS
ARE BLOWN APART, THE
FRESHER THE GROWTH.

SARAH WILSON

Self-acceptance in action

Much like our 'I'll be happy/confident when ...' stories, our 'I'll accept myself when ...' narratives are often based on a feeling of lack or scarcity. They carry with them the belief that right here, right now, I am not enough, I need to be more (patient, kind, interesting, motivated, driven, healthy etc.).

When our actions stem from this place of not enoughness, we end up doing things for the wrong reasons. Desperate to be accepted (by others and ourselves), we get swept into the tide of perfectionism, people-pleasing, or procrastination. We become stressed, burnt-out, or resentful. We make decisions that aren't aligned with our values and who we want to be.

For example:

- The parent who feels unsure of themselves so agrees to join the school committee (even though they are already over-scheduled) in the hope that they will be accepted by this community. Instead of feeling included, they end up feeling stressed and resentful of this new responsibility, tired, and spread too thin.
- The younger person who wants to get fit and healthy but feels like they 'should' go out drinking and dancing with their friends in order to be accepted. They wake the next day feeling tired and disappointed in themselves.
- The staff member who worries they aren't qualified enough so works until late at night to ensure their part of the work project is perfect. When they receive positive feedback on their contribution, they don't feel satisfied as the feeling of not being enough is still there under the surface.

- The person who has an idea for a small business but is worried people will think it's silly or that they aren't qualified or experienced enough. Consumed by what others will think of them, this person gets caught in cycles of procrastination and never makes their dream a reality.

In contrast, when our actions come from a deep belief that we are already enough, we make better decisions. We learn to act in ways that are sustainable and more representative of our values and goals.

For example:

- The parent who is asked to join the school committee but declines as they know this increased responsibility will put pressure on their family and detract from time with their kids.
- The younger person on a health quest who declines a big night out with their friends and wakes in the morning feeling fresh and proud of themselves for honouring what's important to them.
- The staff member who notices when they are caught in cycles of perfectionism and people-pleasing and offers themselves a supportive phrase like, 'You've done enough, it's time to switch off from work.'
- The person keen to start their own small business who notices the fear of being judged but stands strong, willing to chase their dreams, even if it feels uncomfortable.

Each day we make big and small decisions. Learning to take a moment to pause and ensure that your actions are tethered to an inner belief that you are enough is an important aspect of redefining happiness. So how can you do this on a day-to-day basis?

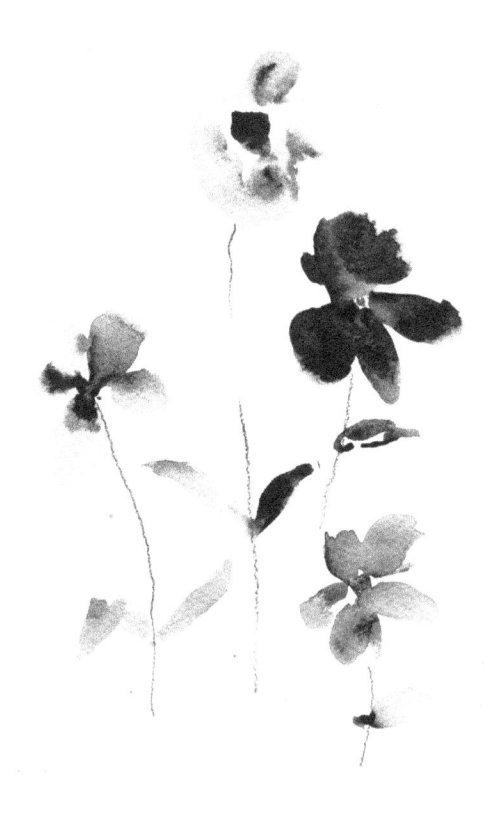

You might remember how, in the perspective pathway, we practiced moving from fear to love by learning to connect with our inner compass. We can use this inner compass here too — allowing it to guide us away from insecurity and self-doubt towards enoughness. Or if you prefer: away from scarcity towards abundance, or from self-resistance to self-acceptance. This practice includes pausing before we make decisions, inviting in a moment of self-acceptance, and then acting from this more whole and authentic place. When we do this, we connect with our natural wellspring of inner motivation and drive.

EXERCISE: YOUR INNER COMPASS (PART TWO)

Try this practice when you need to make a decision.

Begin by taking three deep breaths. Bring a question or situation to mind, something you would like guidance on.

Acknowledge how you are feeling in relation to this question or situation. Notice any subtle expressions of insecurity or resistance. Notice how this feels in your body, maybe like a heaviness or an ache.

As best you can, allow whatever is here to be as it is. You don't need to push it away. But also, you don't need to get pulled in. Just breathe.

Invite in a moment of self-acceptance. Repeat silently in your mind:

Right here, right now, I am enough. I accept myself exactly as I am.

Allow this energy of acceptance to relax your body, to soften you.

Imagine you are holding a compass that has two directions: resistance/insecurity and self-acceptance.

In your own time, move the compass so that it points you in the direction of self- acceptance.

Ask yourself these two questions:

If I believed in myself, how would I move forward?

If I trusted that I was already enough, what is the first action I would take?

Really imagine yourself thinking, feeling, and acting in this way.

Take a deep breath. Smile. You just learnt to calibrate your actions towards greater authenticity and happiness.

Remember, you don't need to do this exercise sitting down with your eyes closed, you can do it anywhere, anytime you need to make a decision that's grounded in self-acceptance.

Walking towards acceptance (and happiness) will be different for each of us — and that's how it should be. I want you to realise, as you arrive at the end of this book, that you can make your own rules and find your own meaning. You can create a life you're incredibly proud of, in spite of (or because of) the challenges you have faced. It all begins with acceptance, even if just for a moment at a time.

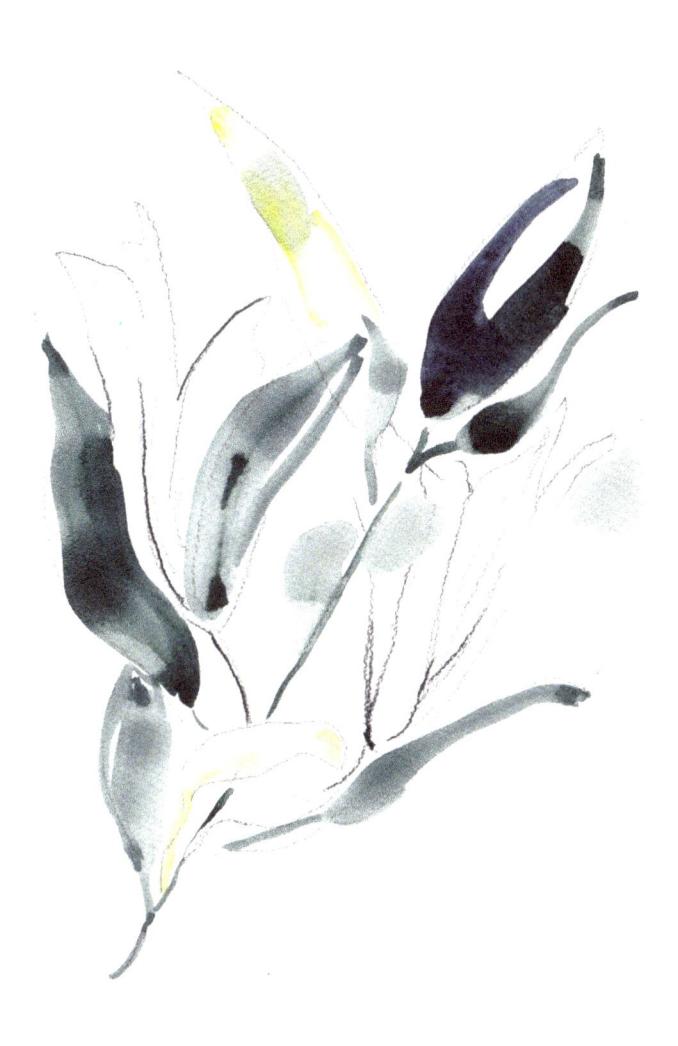

EXERCISE: DARE TO IMAGINE

Focus on how your chest expands in all directions: front, side, and back expanding on each inhale.

Imagine that with each breath you are waking your heart.

Notice any feelings of warmth or ease.

Ask yourself one or both of these questions:

What would my life look and feel like if I accepted myself exactly as I am?

How would I feel if I accepted my life just as it is, right here, right now?

You don't need to have an answer, it's enough just to stay with the question.

Rest in this space of imagination, freedom, and possibility for at least five breaths.

Notice any changes in your physical body (relaxation, softening, lightness).

Notice any changes in your heart (emotions, perspective, outlook).

Ask yourself:

What would I do more of?

What would I let go?

Breathe deep into this moment of possibility. Trust that it is altering your inner landscape and creating space for greater acceptance and freedom in your future.

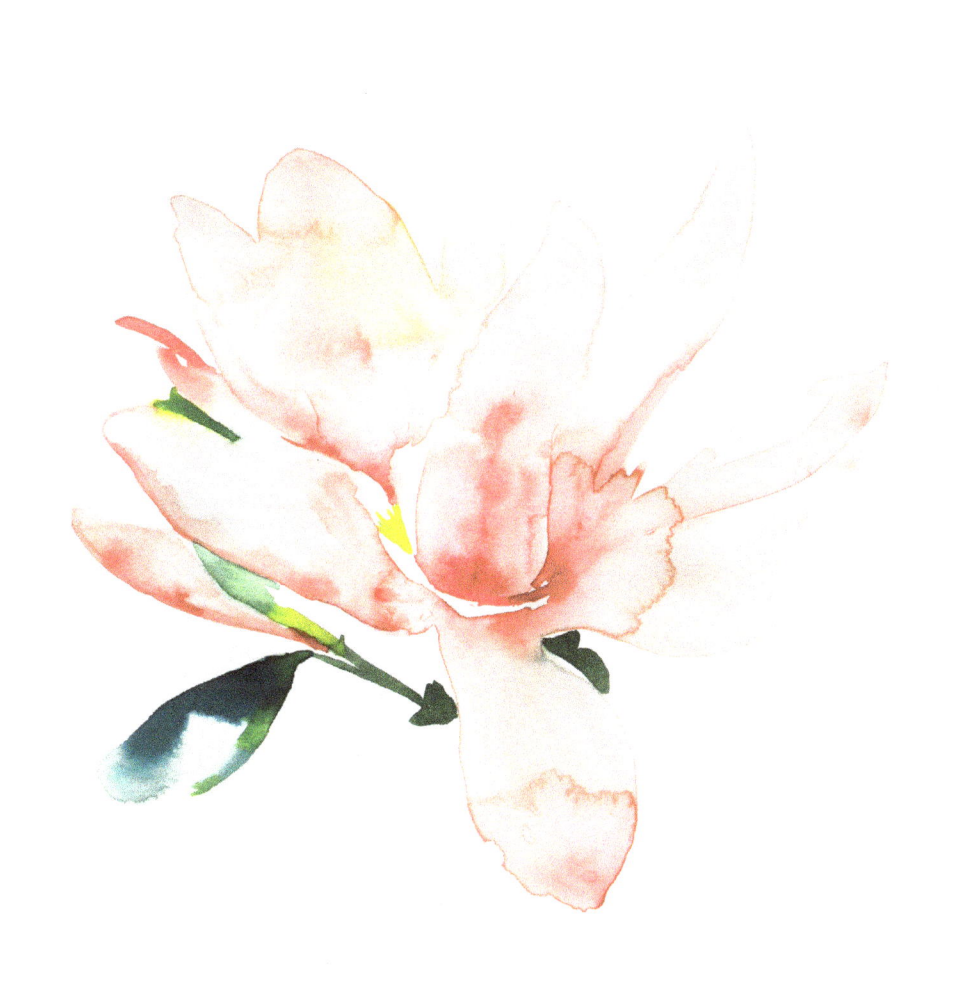

EPILOGUE

Feeling safe in the unknown

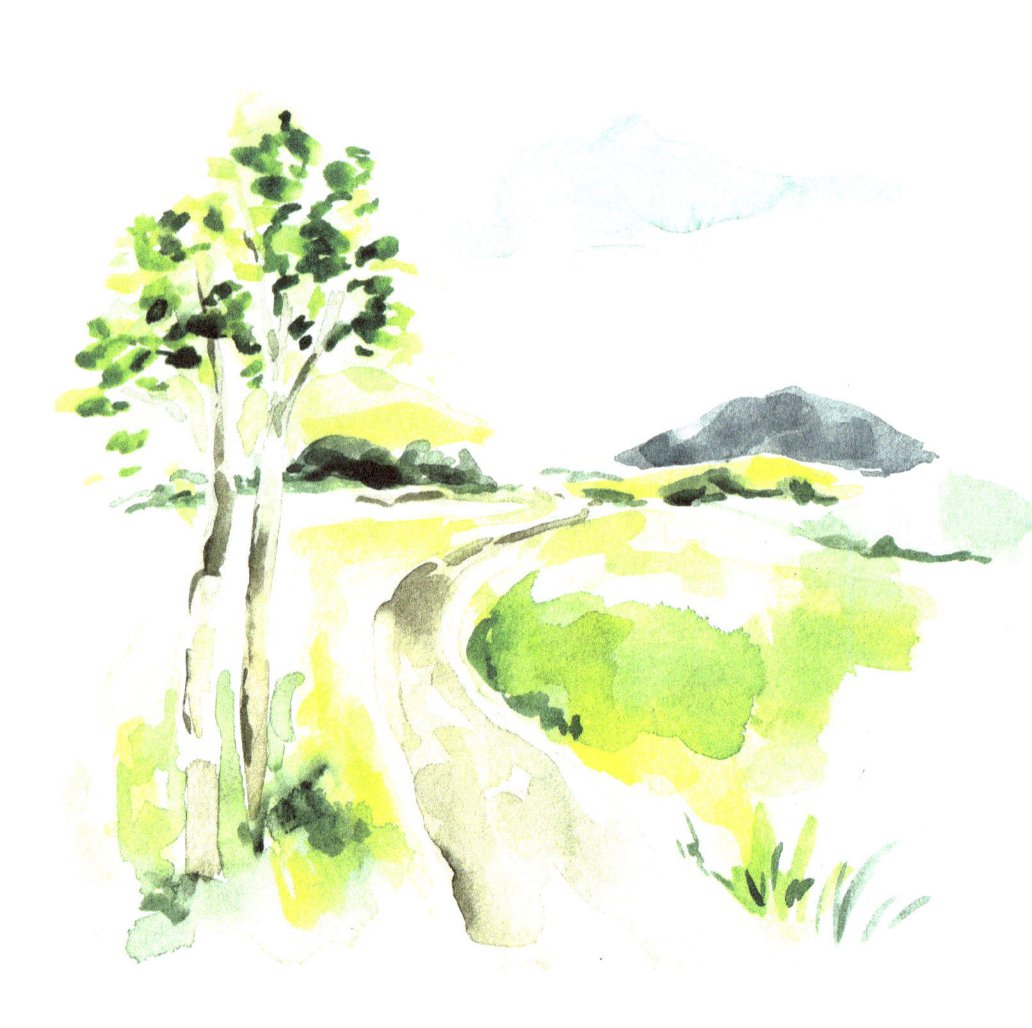

EPILOGUE

Learn to hold your entire experience lightly, with a sense of curiosity, compassion and humour.

Starting to write a book is no small feat, but finishing a book can be even more challenging. As I sat down to type the final pages, I found myself wondering: *What do you, the reader, want to hear? What ending do you really want? How can I make sure that what I've shared has an impact and makes a difference?*

Like a 'good student', I sat with these questions and offered them my warm-hearted curiosity. I soon discovered an undercurrent of fear sitting beneath my creativity. I knew, without a doubt, what was really causing me to question what to write in these final pages. The real question on my mind and heart: *Will my readers be disappointed (in me, this book or my ten pathways framework) if I share with them my truth: that I still experience pain?*

As I write this, I still have the condition which inspired my journey to redefine happiness all those years ago. I am not 'cured'. There hasn't been a moment where, to the amazement of my doctors, my condition disappeared.

However, I have found my own miracle ending, despite the pain I still experience. If I spend the rest of my life in some degree of pain, I know I will be okay — far better than okay. Pain cannot take away my happiness. Knowing this is both empowering and deeply comforting.

Even the doubt I've felt as I write these final chapters has been a gift in itself. I've smiled at how many times writing this book has offered me opportunities for honesty, vulnerability, and healing.

Writing this final chapter, I was reminded of a question a student asked me in my online course, *Breaking the Cycle of Chronic Pain*.

> Why aren't you teaching people how to break free from the pain all together? Don't you believe that it's possible to be totally cured?

As with all the questions I've been asked by students over the years, I remember feeling grateful for the opportunity to reflect, and ultimately, become even more clear in my beliefs and values. My response sounded something like this:

> It's not my role to take people's pain away or to convince people that they can be cured. I'm not here to contribute to any form of striving or chasing. I'm here to help people let go of their resistance, and instead, understand their pain in new and liberating ways.
> My role is to help people sit with their pain with such curiosity, courage, and compassion that it transforms, almost into something beautiful. For me, my pain serves to guide me home, time and time again, to what really matters. It is my hope that each of my students receive the unique gifts held within their experience of pain. Then, and only then, will healing be possible.

So here I am. Honest. Trusting. Hopeful. Sharing with you my version of healed — my happy ending. I still have episodes of pain, but I don't suffer from these experiences. Instead, I listen deeply. I feel grateful. I return home: to the wisdom of my body and my heart, and to an abiding sense that I am safe to surrender into the natural flow of life.

MY PAIN GUIDES ME
HOME TO WHAT REALLY
MATTERS. IT IS MY HOPE
THAT YOU WILL LEARN
TO ACCESS THE WISDOM
HELD WITHIN YOUR PAIN
IN YOUR OWN
UNIQUE WAY.

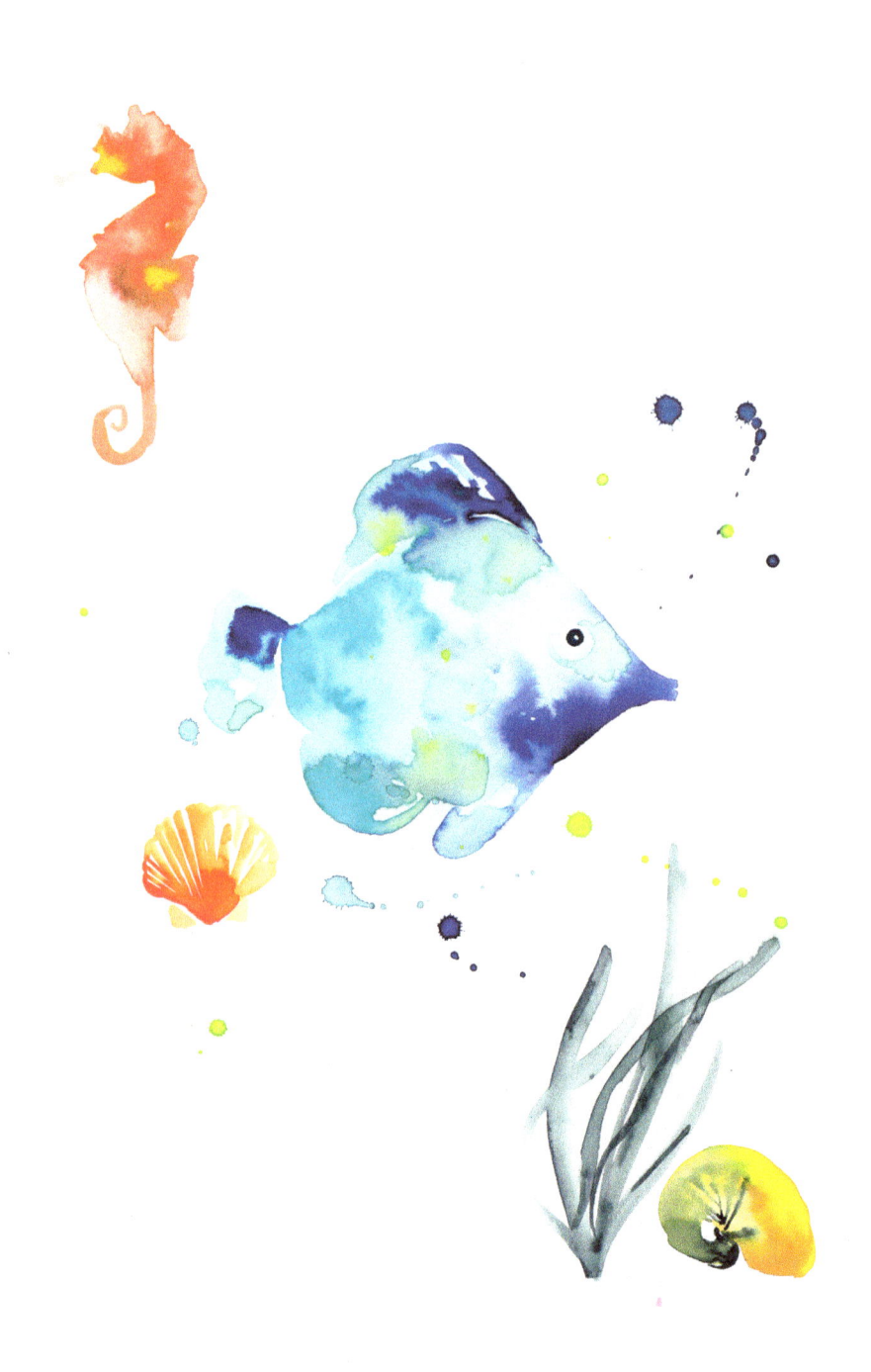

Whilst this version of healed will never make the headlines in our quick-fix, fad-driven world, it's my hope that this more honest and grounded perspective will offer you reassurance. May it remind you that setbacks, challenges, grief, and pain are all natural parts of life. May it encourage you to be with your scars, both old and new, with warm-hearted curiosity. In the act of welcoming these shadows, may you be rewarded with a life that feels more vibrant and meaningful.

Don't forget your travel companions — curiosity, compassion, and a sense of humour

Shortly after the idea for this book came to me, I went stand-up paddleboarding for the first time with a friend. The experience felt extraordinary for two reasons. Firstly, our city was in its sixth pandemic lockdown so, between work and homeschooling, it felt amazing to use our allocated one hour for exercise in such a beautiful way. Secondly, it had been years since I'd dared to move my body in such a physical way.

As we paddled out on this afternoon in spring, the light was gentle, the bay was perfectly still, and the water crystal clear. I said to my friend, 'This feels like something *other* people do.' She smiled and responded, 'It feels like something a holiday me would do.' We laughed and continued paddling, a shared sense of joy washing over us like the tide washes over the sand.

Jellyfish and fiddler rays swam beneath us. A pod of dolphins played around us. And of course, these intelligent animals had a message for me — to open to more joy and creativity.

That night, as I lay in bed, I noticed with both surprise and delight that I wasn't in any physical pain. It felt like a miracle. I remember thinking: *I've done it. I've finally solved the mystery that is my chronic pain. Awe and wonder make my pain disappear!*

Energised by this liberating idea, my mind immediately went off in all directions. I imagined moving my desk and computer outside, eating alfresco every day, and riding my bike everywhere. I was ready to paint all the corners of my life with the colours of awe and wonder.

I lay in bed feeling proud of myself for all the years of doing the deep inner work. This moment of insight felt like a reward for the courage I'd shown in sitting with my pain and listening to what it was trying to teach me. If I'm totally honest, accompanying this pride and satisfaction was a hint of smugness. I'd done what no doctor could do, I'd found my own cure for this mysterious condition. I'd cracked the fibromyalgia code!

The next morning, I woke up in more pain than I had experienced in years.

You would imagine that I'd be disappointed, even crushed. But to my surprise, I didn't feel despondent at all. Nor did I feel foolish or self-critical for my light-bulb moment the night before, that had since lost its luminosity. Instead, I laughed. The type of laugh that bubbles up from deep in your belly and feels like a huge release.

I got out of bed, body riddled with pain, realising once again that our happy endings aren't about finally making sense of it all or getting what we want (or think we deserve). Instead, real happiness is about feeling safe in the mystery and the unknown. It includes learning to hold our entire experience lightly, with a sense of curiosity, compassion, and humour.

Right now, I'm accepting of the resistance I'm feeling towards publishing this book. I'm observing, with curiosity, the voice which says: *Who are you to share your story?* I'm able to smile at this voice because I know thoughts are not facts and that I can trust in the process.

I'm also using my inner compass to reorientate my awareness away from doubt (fear), towards my desire to help others (love). I'm trusting once again that our discomfort is an opportunity to discover more about ourselves and to step fully into the miracle of living each day on our precious planet Earth.

I don't know what challenges you may face in the future, but I trust that if you come back to this ten pathway framework, it will help you face them with softness, acceptance, and even amazement. And I trust the same will be true for me — even with pain as my companion.

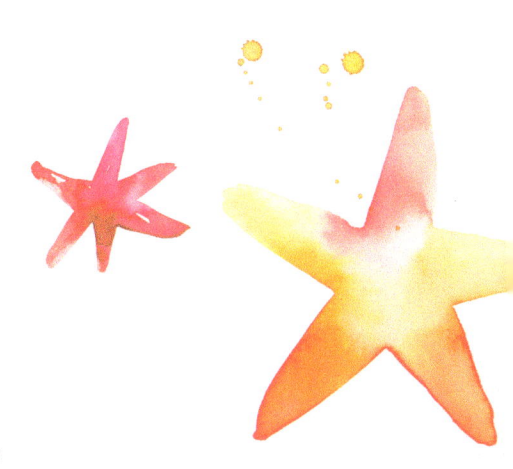

REFERENCES

PATHWAY 1: AWARENESS

Killingsworth, M. and Gilbert, D. T. 2010, 'A wandering mind is an unhappy mind', *Science,* Vol. 330 no. 6006

PATHWAY 2: COMPASSION

The Arrow Sallatha Sutta, SN 36:6 https://www.dhammatalks.org/suttas/SN/SN36_6.html

Neff, K. 2015, *Self-Compassion, The Proven Power of Being Kind to Yourself*

Neff, K. and Germer, C. 2018, *The Mindful Self-Compassion Workbook*

Suzuki, S. 2011, *Zen Mind, Beginner's Mind: Informal Talks on Zen Meditation and Practice*

Moore, T. 2021, *Captain Tom's Life Lessons*

The HeartMath Institute, 2016, *Science of the Heart, Vol. 2*

PATHWAY 3: PERSPECTIVE

White, F. 2014, *The Overview Effect: Space Exploration and Human Evolution*

Darnall, B. 2016, *The Opioid-Free Pain Relief Kit: 10 Simple Steps to Ease Your Pain*

Darnall, B. 2018, *Psychological Treatment for Patients with Chronic Pain*

Herriott, A., Herriott, J., Obysseus, T. 2016, *The Wonder Method: Energy Healing and the Art of Awakening Through Wonder*

Einstein, A. 1931, *Living Philosophies*

Allen, S. 2018, 'The Science of Awe', Prepared by The Greater Good Science Center at CU Berkeley, https://ggsc.berkeley.edu/images/uploads/GGSC-JTF_White_Paper-Awe_FINAL.pdf

Elkins, D. N. 2001, 'Reflections on Mystery and Awe', Elkins, D. N. 2001, *The Psychotherapy Patient,* Vol.11

PATHWAY 4: GRATITUDE

Sacks. O. 2015, *Gratitude*

Emmons, R. A. *Thanks! How the New Science of Gratitude Can Make You Happier*

Seneca, L 2021, *Letters from a Stoic*

PATHWAY 5: CALM

Neff, K., and Germer, C., 'The Transformative Effects of Mindful Self-Compassion' January 29, 2019, Well-Being (mindful.org)

Malouf, D. 2011, The Happy Life, *The Quarterly Essays,* QE41, March

PATHWAY 6: CONNECTION

Baird, J. 2020, *Phosphorescence*

The Indigenous Weather Knowledge website, http://www.bom.gov.au/iwk/index.shtml

Tewari, B. 2019, 'Vedic Seasons', *Prakriti*, February 18, 2019

Nhat Hanh, T. 2015, *The Heart of the Buddha's Teachings*

PATHWAY 7: PURPOSE

Csikszentmihalyi, M. 1998, *Finding Flow: The Psychology of Engagement With Everyday Life*

Hanson, R. 'Honoring Your Childhood Dreams' *Being Well Podcast*, Season 2, Episode 44

PATHWAY 8: VITALITY

Nhat Hanh, T. 2019, *Present Moment, Wonderful Moment*

Brown, B. 2021, *Daring Greatly*

PATHWAY 9: CONFIDENCE

Hanson, R. 2018, *Resilient*

PATHWAY 10: ACCEPTANCE

Tedeschi, R. G., Shakespeare-Finch, J., Taku, K., and Calhoun, L. G., 2018, *Posttraumatic Growth*

Wilson, S. 2017, *First, We Make The Beast Beautiful*

Loft, P. The Gentle Osteopath, https://www.gentleosteopath.com.au/

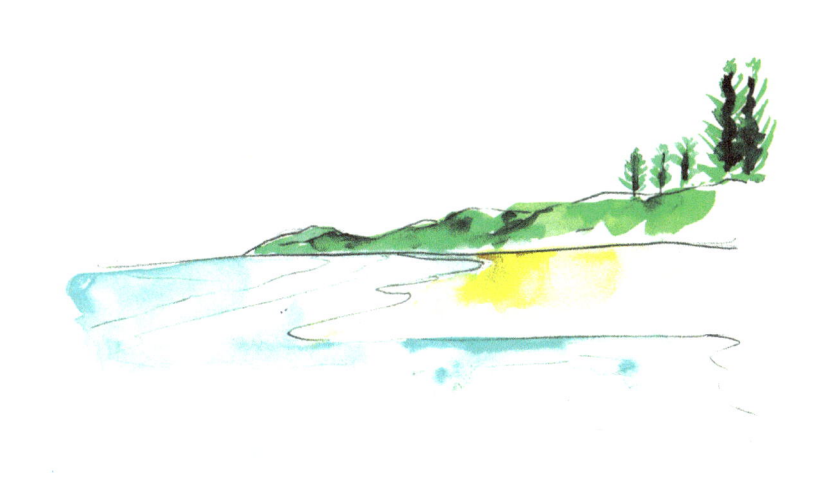

ACKNOWLEDGEMENTS

Thank you to my mum, dad, brother, and sister for knowing and loving me the longest. To my husband, Andrew, and my boys, Tom, Gabe, and Dash, for encouraging me (in their own unique ways), for making me laugh when I least expect it and for offering me the best reason to be present.

Thank you to my international meditation community who share with me their inner worlds. Each of your stories has helped me understand more fully the shared joys and challenges of being human.

To all my teachers: the spiritual masters, the neuroscientists, and the regular people who show me through their actions how courageous and compassionate we can be. And of course, to all the animals who have offered me wisdom along the way.

To my editor, Amy Molloy, who offered both her intellect and her heart to the process of editing my book. Thank you for helping me find my writer's voice (very different to my meditation voice apparently!) and for holding me and this book during my moments of vulnerability.

To my publisher, Karen McDermott, who read one chapter and said 'yes'. It's a pleasure to work with someone who makes decisions as quickly as I do.

Finally, this book is so much more than my words. Sending out my gratitude to Sarah and Bree Hankinson, the creative sisters who illustrated and designed this book respectively. Both these women participated in some of my first meditation classes. Given how much I enjoy synchronicity, it feels wonderful to have taken our shared love of 'seeing the beauty in the ordinary everyday moments' to the next level when collaborating on this book.

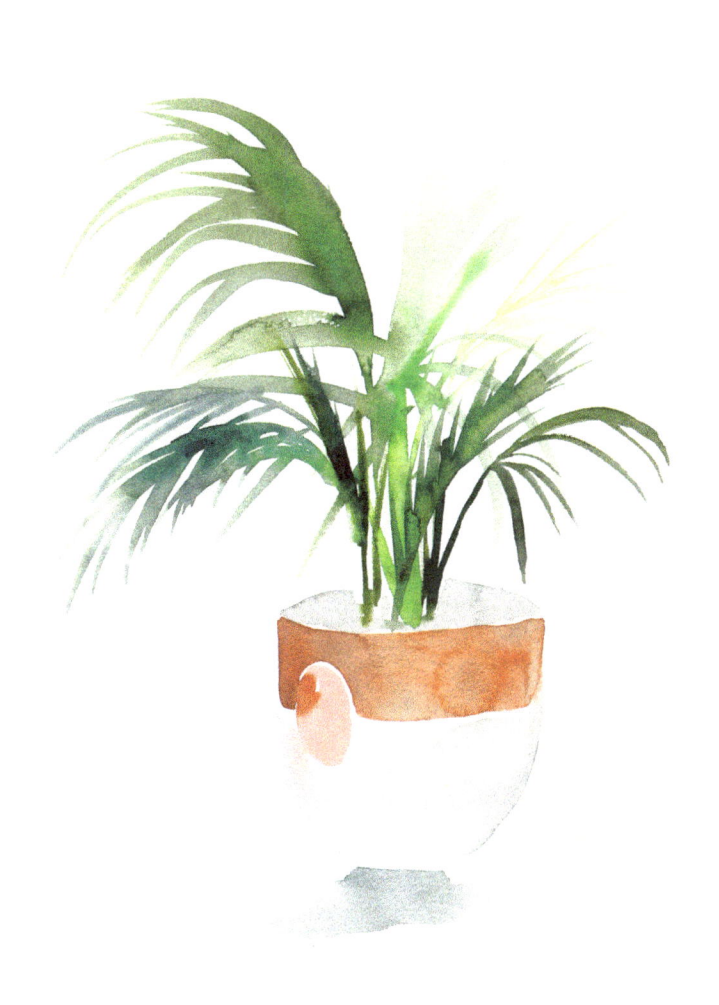

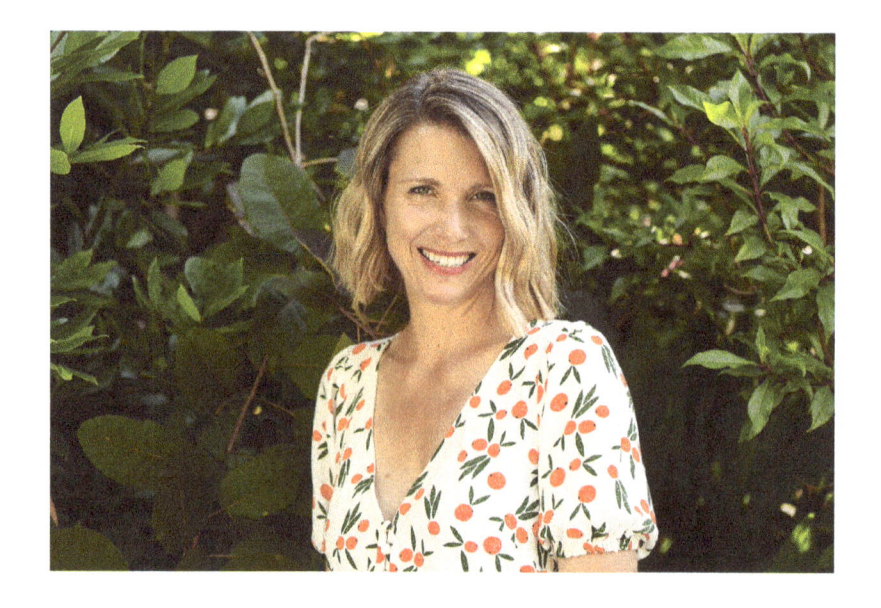

Fleur Chambers is a multi-award-winning, internationally recognised meditation teacher and creator of *The Happy Habit* app. Her offerings have been downloaded two million times in over forty countries. Proceeds from all Fleur's projects go towards grassroots projects that tackle poverty in some of the world's poorest communities. Her work, and your participation, are powerful reminders that we can improve our own lives and contribute to the world in positive ways — one breath at a time.

Fleur lives near the beach in Melbourne, with her husband, three boys, and dog Lucky.

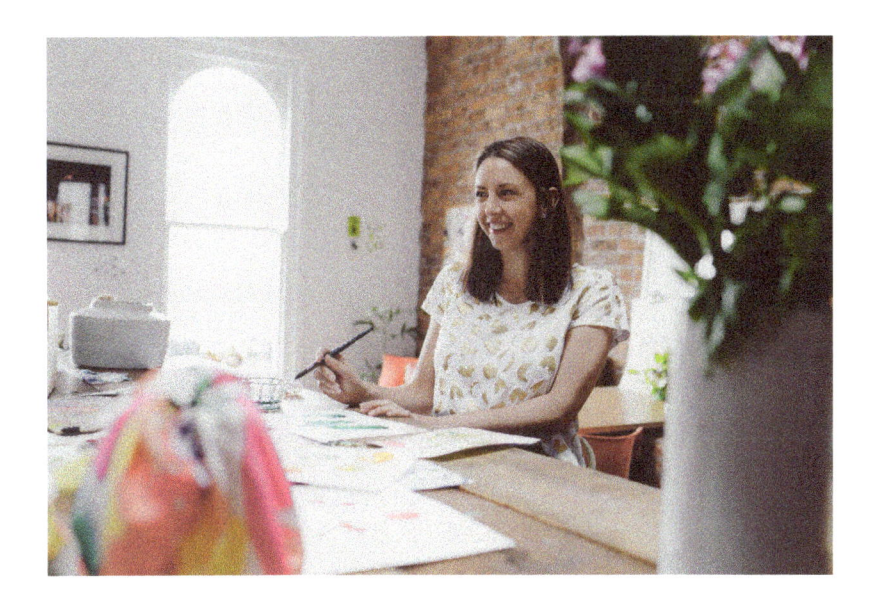

Illustrator Sarah Hankinson, born, raised, and currently residing in Melbourne, Australia, studied both graphic design and fine art before discovering her love of illustration, graduating in 2004. Currently, Sarah combines her freelance illustrating career, along with being a mum of two small boys, and other creative pursuits such as managing The Windsor Workshop co-working studio in Melbourne's south.

Having spent years capturing the essence of everyday moments through her illustrations, Sarah enjoyed bringing this sense of mindfulness and presence into her life as a mother.

Lightning Source UK Ltd.
Milton Keynes UK
UKHW022119230223
417533UK00012B/207